Unmarried Without Children

A Journey to Marriage and Motherhood

By: Alisha J.

"Unmarried Without Children: A Journey to Marriage and Motherhood" Copyright © 2023 (Alisha J.)

ISBN: 979-8-9869787-1-0

EBOOK ISBN: 979-8-9869787-3-4

All rights reserved. No part of this book may be reproduced, stored in a retrieval system, or transmitted in any form or by any means, electronic, mechanical, recording, or otherwise without written permission from the author.

Scripture quotations marked "KJV" are taken from the Holy Bible, King James Version (Public Domain).

Scripture quotations marked "AMP" are taken from the Amplified® Bible, Copyright © 1954, 1958, 1962, 1964, 1965, 1987 by The Lockman Foundation. Used by permission.

Scripture quotations marked (NLT) are taken from the Holy Bible, New Living Translation, copyright © 1996, 2004, 2007 by Tyndale House Foundation. Used by permission of Tyndale House Publishers, Inc., Carol Stream, Illinois 60188. All rights reserved.

Published by: New Voice Books LLC

Contact number: 972-637-3321

Website: nvpublishingco.com

Edited by: Speak Write Play, LLC and New Voice Books, LLC

Dedication

I dedicate this book to my mother who birthed me, Alfreda Starks Blanding; the mother who raised me, Veta Williams Blanding; and my father, Gerard Blanding Sr., who was both my mother and father for a season. I thank God for giving them the courage, insight, and wisdom to raise me into the woman I am today.

I'd like to dedicate this book to my future husband, whom I have prayed for and loved before manifesting in my life. I know that God has ordained us to be together at a specific time for a specific purpose, and I know you are also praying for me.

To my beautiful future children. As I prepare and pray for you, I am so excited about meeting and raising you, with your father, to be God-fearing, well-rounded individuals. I look forward to cultivating the gifts that God will bless you with and encouraging your talents as you grow into mature adults. I already love you and can't wait to meet you.

Foreword

Waiting is hard. It doesn't matter if you're waiting to get married, have a baby or to check out in one of Walmart's long lines. In a fast-paced world where everything is readily accessible, there is nothing easy about having to wait.

In the past 10+ years of trying to have a baby, I've learned first-hand how hard it is to be in a season of waiting. It's isolating, nerve wrecking, and mentally exhausting. Let's just say that waiting on your heart's desire can be an emotional rollercoaster full of twists and turns. But even with all the inner turmoil that can come with waiting, I have also experienced God's unfailing love and sweet grace during the process. At times it was as if God was saying "Daughter, I know this is hard. But I'm right here with you".

I met Alisha through a mutual friend during that time in my life when God began to consistently show me that He was with me. Her bubbly personality coupled with her amazing story has inspired me beyond measure. Being in a dual waiting season is no easy feat. I imagine it takes great faith and tenacity to wait on your God-ordained husband while going through fertility issues at the same time. But Alisha has proven that it can be done when you're surrounded by people who genuinely love and support you.

In this book, Alisha invites you to walk a mile in her shoes by taking you through her journey of waiting step-by-step. It won't make you feel like you're on the outside looking in, but instead it'll feel like you were right there with her. Throughout this book you'll want to laugh, cry and ask God "WHY!?". In a nutshell, you'll get an in-depth lesson of how real the struggle can be, but you'll also be reminded of how loving and faithful God is.

- *Geri Alicea*

Founder of Womb Prep

Acknowledgements

I'd like to acknowledge my parents, all my friends and family members who are a part of my village, and the members of the Womb Prep Facebook Group. Your love, consistent nudging, prayers, and continued support have motivated me to write this book. I would also like to acknowledge Geri Alicea and thank her for contributing to my first book, for being an inspiration, and for pouring into my life.

Introduction

To every thing there is a season, and a time to every purpose under the heaven.

–*Ecclesiastes 3:1 (KJV)*

As a little girl, I would play dress up in my mother's wedding dress, dreaming of the day I would walk down the aisle toward my handsome groom. I would spend countless hours pretending that my baby dolls were my real babies, ensuring they were well-fed, entertained, changed, and well-rested. These were my goals:

- Go to college.

- Get married.

- Have three children.

- Have a distinguished career.

It seemed cut and dry when I was little, but life would prove that God's plans were different than mine.

Of these goals, I have been able to complete my college education. I am now settling into my career in implementation management and entrepreneurship. Still, there are two areas in my life that, for a season, I felt I was failing to accomplish, *marriage and motherhood*.

I have spent many nights crying to God, asking Him to send me my husband, begging Him to prepare me to be a wife, and getting frustrated when asked to be a bridesmaid in yet another wedding while still waiting for God to manifest *my* husband.

Just like the kissing nursery rhyme we used to sing as children instructed us, *first comes love, then comes marriage, then comes the baby in the baby carriage*; I desired to do things God's way, so I did all that I could do to set myself up for success in becoming a wife—including serial dating, hiring a wife preparation coach, vowing celibacy, serving in the church, reading multiple books on the subject of how to attract your spouse, and fasting and praying. But to no avail.

Year after year, I watched friends and family members get married. I bought multiple bridesmaid dresses, attended and hosted bridal showers, and smiled through photos, but wondering *God, what about me? When will it be my turn?* I began to feel like the man at the pool at Bethesda[1].

Then in 2018, I noticed something wasn't quite right with my health. I was having extreme hot flashes more often than I had in the past. My body was changing, and I wasn't sure what to make of it. My cycles were irregular and heavier, I had night sweats, and my mood swings were extreme. *I thought, surely this cannot be menopause; I'm only thirty-four.*

After seeking answers from my doctors, they informed me that I was perimenopausal and experiencing pre-ovarian failure. I was shocked, and my faith in God wavered. This was the first time I experienced challenges I didn't have a solution for and couldn't fix.

Faced with delays in becoming married and fertility challenges, I have had to learn how to navigate through my thoughts, feelings, fears, and faith. Fortunately, I am blessed enough to go through this journey with loving friends, family, and a tribe of women who can relate.

---

[1] John 5: 1 – 6 (NLT).

Unmarried Without Children is God-inspired to share my story with every working, wonderful, and whimsical woman who is wondering whether God has forgotten about her. She may be asking God why her season of being unmarried and childless is lasting so long. Or she may be saying, "Is my Heavenly Father even listening to my prayers for marriage and motherhood?"

Through this book, my desire is to encourage you to find hope again and be reminded of God's faithfulness. This book is a testament to God's faithfulness and a manifestation of His prophetic word that He revealed to one of my close friends in a dream.

I genuinely believe that God will grant you the desires of your heart, and I pray that after reading this book, you will believe again. Indeed, if God said it, it *will* come to pass.

Table of Contents

Chapter 1 – In the Beginning

Chapter 2 – The Dating Game

Chapter 3 – The Diagnosis

Chapter 4 – The Blame Game

Chapter 5 – The Seven Stages of Grief

Chapter 6 – Purpose in My Pain

Chapter 7 – The Village

Chapter 8 – Don't Put Your Eggs in One Basket

Chapter 1
In the Beginning

Thank you for making me so wonderfully complex! Your workmanship is marvelous—how well I know it. You watched me as I was being formed in utter seclusion, as I was woven together in the dark of the womb. You saw me before I was born. Every day of my life was recorded in your book. Every moment was laid out before a single day had passed.

–Psalm 139:14-16 (NLT)

It was all a dream. I used to play with Barbies dolls and dress up in wedding dresses as a little girl. I dreamed of my big day, imagining myself walking down the aisle and being escorted by father. My dress was big, white, and poofy covered in rhinestones and crystals as I walked toward my fiancé, beaming with pride. I always dreamed of the wedding and the three kids we would have. Our eldest, a boy, and our twins, one boy and one girl. I even had the names chosen.

I mean, I was ready, ready. I had it all planned out. At twenty-five, I was going to be married. At twenty-seven, my firstborn would arrive, and by thirty, I would have twins. But God looked at my plans and laughed. I remember the day when He said to me, "I have need of you." I didn't understand what He meant then, but I understand it better now. I must admit, I never thought this would happen to me.

I never thought in a million years that I would be dealing with infertility. Infertility is not a respecter of persons. It doesn't consider your skin color, socioeconomic status, or cultural background; it can affect any woman at any age and at any time.

During my journey, I learned that girls as young as seventeen years old deal with infertility. I was thirty-four years old when I found out that my chances of becoming a mother—my lifelong dream—were slim to none.

I cried and questioned God. I yelled and screamed. I even had adult temper tantrums because I thought God wasn't treating me fairly. I often asked God, "Why her and not me?" Even though I didn't understand it, and in the midst of my pain and anguish, I still had faith that God would perform a miracle in my life. But I made three mistakes.

As I mentioned earlier, I had it all mapped out. I wasn't sure where my family would live, but I knew we would either be middle class or wealthy. I would ride off into the sunset in my SUV. But God has a funny way of interrupting our plans. My timeline, my perception of how my body functioned biologically, and my ignorance around fertility and infertility had me feeling lost and confused for a time. After reading this book, my hope is that you will avoid making the three mistakes.

My first mistake was thinking I had more time. I thought that my delay in marriage wouldn't be an issue because my maternal grandmother was in her forties when she had her fourteenth child. So, in my mind, genetics had me believing that I, too, could have children well into my forties. I had a monthly cycle (PMS included). I was healthy and young. That's all I needed to be a mother, right? Boy, was I wrong.

Now, don't be mistaken. I was aware of the risks that accompanied having children in my forties, such as a higher probability of having children with Down syndrome and other genetic disorders, but that didn't worry me. The course that

God had me on proved to be far from the life I had imagined for myself. I was settled in my mind to be content with it as long as I was married and had a child by the time, I was forty. In 2 Peter 3:8 it says, "But do not forget this one thing, dear friends: With the Lord a day is like a thousand years, and a thousand years are like a day" (NIV). I guess I just forgot that God didn't move according to my timelines nor my demands.

My second mistake was being ignorant about how biology works. I wasn't taught about menopause, polycystic ovary syndrome (PCOS), fibroids, or endometriosis. I remember being in sex ed class in middle school and watching how the sperm traveled to fertilize the egg. I learned that during gestation, if the embryo is female, she will be born with all the eggs she will ever have in her entire lifetime. I didn't know what that meant as far as childbearing.

As I went further into the research about the female embryo, I learned about the egg reserve. Throughout a female's lifetime, eggs are continuously released due to her cycle or for various other reasons. Once those eggs are gone, the female is unable to regenerate new eggs. Since eggs are not regenerated, the egg reserve eventually becomes depleted. Once this happens, a female begins to go through menopause, or a period of 365 days without having a cycle. Outside of a miracle from God, a female will have to consider getting an egg donor if she has a healthy uterus and desires to have a child.

My third mistake was not knowing my fertility options earlier in life. I'd moved through life completely in the dark until I learned that I was going through perimenopause at an age younger than expected. No man or woman knows the day nor the hour when they will be married or whether becoming a parent would be simple or more challenging compared to others. I know I am taking Matthew 24:36 out of context, but it is so true. I had no clue when I would be married, and my plan was not to be well into my thirties and still single. What's crazy is that God had been trying to tell me for years that my journey to motherhood would be challenging.

He told me through the Holy Spirit, dreams, and even people who barely knew me. My first revelation came almost ten years ago when I was sitting in my room and faintly heard the Holy Spirit whisper, "Satan is trying to block your seed because he knows what your seed will do to his kingdom." Immediately, I went into warfare mode and began declaring blessings over my family, decreeing that Satan had no dominion or power over us and that my spouse would manifest on time. But as time went on, my prayers wavered, and I began to lose hope that God was even listening to me. This began to make me wonder about certain decisions I made on my journey that could have led to me having a child outside of marriage, but we'll talk about that later.

The second time God tried to inform me about my unconventional path to motherhood came in a dream in 2017. I was lying in the birthing position in my dream. Although it may sound strange, I could physically feel my body contorting to the position as well. In my dream, I saw the forms of three babies. As the first child was born, a hand appeared and snatched it away.

Then, the baby transitioned from a human form into a shadow. I felt the baby leaving me. The same happened with the second baby. However, with the third baby, as I was birthing it, I could only see its arm. And its hand was a fist. Then, I saw the baby's face. This baby was not snatched away and didn't fade into a shadow. I woke up after that.

I had no clue what God was trying to say to me at the time, so I went to see a friend who interpreted dreams. After telling her my dream, she gave me a response that came from the Book of Revelation. In my spirit, I didn't believe her interpretation was correct. Also, I didn't consult God further about the matter, so like before, I went on about my business. During that same year, I had another prophetic dream. In case you haven't picked up on it by now, God speaks to me through dreams.

But during these seasons in my life, I wasn't fully aware of the extent of the power behind my dreams. This time, I dreamt of a little four or five-year-old chocolate-skinned boy who looked and felt real. He must have been my son because I felt a love for him like I had never felt for any human before. It was unconditional love. I was so in love with this little boy.

When I woke up, I thanked God that He allowed me to dream about my son. One year after this fantastic dream, I was working for a Fortune 500 company and began fanning myself in a meeting. My coworker asked me how I was doing, and I explained to her that I was having hot flashes. I didn't think anything of it because I regularly had hot flashes during PMS, so it was normal to me. I also told her that my grandmother was forty when she had her last child, so I wasn't worried.

With concern in her voice, she suggested that I freeze my eggs. Not realizing she was trying to help, I shrugged off the suggestion because I thought she was being nosey. I just knew I had time to have children. All my life, all I ever wanted was to be a wife and mother. Even in kindergarten, I had a pretend wedding on the playground and married a little boy named M.C., so these desires have been a part of my life for as long as I can remember.

I suppose my strong desire to be a wife and mother came from losing my biological mother to leukemia when I was six years old. Although it wasn't long after her death before my father remarried, I still had a void in my heart. I felt like something was missing, and I longed to be married. I wanted to start a family of my own. Perhaps it was my way of fixing what I believed broke in me as a child.

I also believe that being a witness to all the strong marriages in my family caused this strong desire to be married. My grandparents were married for over 60 years before my grandfather passed in 2020. My parents have been married for over 30 years. And I have countless aunts and uncles who have been married for years and make it look so effortless and amazing. I must admit, I had a fantastic childhood.

My supernatural mother (Veta), whom I affectionately call "mommy" or "ma" (depending on the need), stepped right in to love and care for me as if she gave birth to me herself. She not only literally saved my life when I almost drowned in

Lake Lanier, but she has been my rock, prayer warrior, and number one supporter since day one. Raising me as a single parent, my father never abandoned me and did the best he could. He made sure I was well-rounded, well-fed, loved, and provided for. I never felt as though there was a lack of love in my life.

My family often went on summer vacation trips. We visited Disney World, Universal Studios, Hilton Head and numerous other Florida beaches. We still go on family vacations to this day. My brother and I went to the best schools, and we lived in safe neighborhoods. Overall, my childhood memories are good, joyous ones. Despite my great upbringing, no amount of love could fill the void of losing my biological mother because I didn't know how to heal from such a loss.

It wasn't just about not having my mother; my innocence was lost, too. I struggled to figure out who I was during my adolescent years. Perhaps I put way too much pressure on myself to discover who I was at such a young age. I never seemed to fit in, and part of that could have been due to the changes I experienced. I had friends, but I was too black for the white kids and too white for the black kids.

I went from being in a multicultural environment to being one of ten black people (students and staff) in my whole school. During my teenage years, I had several thoughts of suicide. I even made one attempt when I was at an all-time low. Being called by God, innovative, proper, black, a girl, outspoken, and assertive felt like blessings and curses. Not to mention, I felt a lot of pressure to be perfect because I had parents in ministry.

Sometimes, the bullying and pressure were overwhelming, so I tried as much I could to be "Perfect Patty." I would overthink every move I made and study all night long to make all A's. I thought I was always better than everyone and had to be smarter. When I wasn't, I was devastated. One day, after feeling tired of trying to be perfect, I just gave up, well, sort of. It was the night before a final (I believe it was a biology final), and as per usual, I'd procrastinated and waited until the last minute to study.

See, I was good at memorizing information, but I was horrible at retaining it. I would take great notes in class and study just to get an A on a test. But I would forget everything I learned the very next day. I mean, it worked until the night when I decided that I wasn't going to study as hard anymore. Like so many times before, I'd gone upstairs to my room to begin the process of cramming for my biology exam the next morning. I took out the pack of blank note cards and robotically began to copy my well-written notes. After completing this process, which took anywhere from 2–3 hours, I began the reciting the notes out loud. Midway through my ritual, I got tired. Not just sleepy, I got tired of being perfect and pretending to know everything. I was just tired. So, instead of staying up until 3 AM to study, I chose to sleep. I ended up getting my first C, but I still managed to earn an A in the class. My perfectionistic attitude landed me at my dream college, Emory University, but high school senioritis caught up with me.

This was when the death of Perfect Patty began. I didn't study as hard as I used to and made my first failing grades ever in my life. My career path was to major in chemistry, become a doctor, and discover a cure to cancer. But my will to just relax and have fun overrode my drive for perfection. College introduced something to me that I didn't really have in high school—a social life.

My love for God never changed. I knew I was called to be a minister and still tried to do my best to be a good Christian girl, but college became my time for freedom. I let my guard down more. I had a little too much fun, and my grades reflected that. I finished school, but Perfect Patty didn't graduate college with high honors.

I failed a couple of classes (I failed organic chemistry twice). As a young adult, I recognized that I was broken, hypocritical, and unsure of who I was as a person and in Christ. I realized that my identity had been wrapped up in the opinions of others for years. I'd become stuck in a conditional life, where I believed that if I did things a certain way (i.e., go to college, find a good job, get married, have kids), that this was what would make my life perfect. I didn't realize that I'd discover I was an entrepreneur at heart by seeking God's will for my life.

I thought I needed to have a few more life experiences, like dating and learning about my body, before I would be married and become a mother. I've also wasted so much time comparing my life to others that I wish I could be like US Congresswoman Maxine Waters and reclaim my time. But time is something that we can never get back. I'd been sheltered, to a certain extent, most of my life, so navigating situations as an adult became difficult and overwhelming. I feel like this is what any young adult feels when they're adulting. No one told us life could be *this* challenging.

My parents made it look so easy and like they had all the money in the world. But one day, I woke up and realized this was not the childhood I grew up in—living paycheck to paycheck, getting overdrafts everywhere, and trying to figure out whether I should go back to school (and if so, who was going to pay for it?). I tried to plan a vacation, but then realized I barely had enough to pay rent, start a business, and do everything. I believe that once I accepted the path for my life, I was able to gain a better understanding of who I am in Christ and who Alisha J. really is.

My prayer for you:

Abba, I pray that my dear sister, will have an undistracted devotion to You in her unmarried season. As she continues to pursue her purpose and calling, may You give her peace and strength to be able to accomplish what it is that You have called her to do.

May she believe in her heart that You have made her fearfully and wonderfully (Ps. 139:14 -16) and that in her time of waiting to be a wife and mother, that you will remind her that You are giving her grace and glory and keeping no good thing from her (Ps. 84:11).

I pray that she will be still in Your presence (Ps.37:7) and be assured that all things are working together for her good because she loves you and is called according to Your purpose (Rom. 8:28). In Jesus' name I pray this prayer. Amen.

Chapter 2
The Dating Game

There are three things that amaze me—no, four things that I don't understand: how an eagle glides through the sky, how a snake slithers on a rock, how a ship navigates the ocean, how a man loves a woman.

–Proverbs 30:18-19 (NLT)

Have you ever asked God, "This can't be it"? Where are all the God-fearing men that You created? The ones that are whole, hardworking, and (let's not kid ourselves) handsome? I mean, it seems as though the dating pool has pee in it, right? We're out here pulling out all the stops while it seems as though the men aren't exerting the same effort or aren't on our level. Now, let me be honest, this is not the case with all the men out there.

Sometimes, it's us who mess things up. But it appears as if even with all the tools like apps and matchmakers, we are still having a hard time being found by the one.

I wasn't allowed to date until my junior year of high school. Even though my parents said I could date when I was sixteen, I had to wait a whole year because I turned sixteen in the tenth grade. Of course, I thought this cramped my style because my goal in life was to be married and have kids. Naturally, I had secret crushes and boyfriends throughout elementary and middle school.

When the time finally came for me to have an official boyfriend, it was like the guys I had crushes on did not even look in my direction. And I didn't like the guys who liked me. To add insult to injury, I went to a predominantly white high school. So, the chances of me having a boyfriend were slim to none because the white guys didn't look twice at me—black girl problems. I didn't have my first boyfriend until I was almost seventeen. I wasn't sincerely attracted to him and even felt embarrassed to be seen with him at times.

I think I was so desperate to have a boyfriend back then that I settled for the first guy who gave me attention. And he was, well, I'll let you form your opinion of him. My mother once told me that I only dated him because he had curly hair. I don't think that was the case either. But the longer I stayed with him, the more I tried to figure out why I was with him. At the end of the day, I will say that I have never dated a man that lied so much for no reason at all in my life.

This man would lie just because it was Sunday. For instance, not too long after 9/11, there was another plane crash in the Rockaway Peninsula in Queens, New York. He called me from his home (this was before caller ID became popular) to tell me that he was in New York at the airport and was watching as the paramedics were loading bodies onto the planes. Through tears, he proceeded to tell me that he could smell the aroma of burnt bodies as they were wheeled out. Even now, I am amazed at my naivety.

I am almost embarrassed to reveal that I believed every word he said. He was crying, so it had to be true. This happened in the era when cell phones were not a main means of communication. So, this conversation was held on the landline aka the house phone in my parent's kitchen. As the conversation progressed, my mother noticed the concern on my face and began to ear hustle (listen in on the conversation). At some point, she asked me what was going on, and I explained to her all that he told me. My mother quickly went into mom mode because she knew he was lying about the entire thing. She tried to tell me this, but I didn't listen. And she could tell that I was convinced he was telling me the truth. I know I am not the only one who has had that one boyfriend that she would like to forget. But I digress. Seeing that my mind was made up, my mother asked me to ask him for his mother's number.

Unbeknownst to me, my mother went upstairs and called his mother while we were still chatting about his "traumatic" experience. Soon after giving my mother the number, she requested, I heard a woman's voice in the background yelling at my boyfriend. He quickly hung up, and we broke up soon after that. Turns out, he was at home in his basement, and the voice in the background was his mother's. I don't know what attracted me to this man. I only stayed as long as I did to say I had a boyfriend. Unfortunately, this was a pattern that I have continued to repeat. I am a loyalist to what I want to be loyal to, and I have a bad habit of holding on to things much longer than I need to.

This is more than likely rooted in the issues I have with the abandonment I felt when my mother passed away, but my therapist and I are working through this now. After graduating from college, I found myself trying to handle my newfound freedoms without a care. I was still active in ministry. I sang in the church choir, participated in the dance ministry, and assisted my parents when they started their church. It was like I was living a double life.

Though I was "Alisha the Perfect PK" in church, I was "Alisha Looking for Love in All the Wrong Places" for the rest of the week. I lost my virginity in college (I'll go into more detail about this later). After that door opened, all hell broke loose. But because of my conviction, I did everything but the deed with most of the guys I was involved with or dated. Still, there were times when I slipped up and sinned against God and myself.[2] To avoid this, I stopped dating for a while and submerged myself in ministry, work, and extracurricular activities like acting, doing makeup, and starting my businesses.

"Busy work," as I call it, kept me occupied and made me think I still had time to start a family. I did not realize I needed

---

[2] 1 Cor. 6:18 (NLT).

to heal. I needed to take a good look in the mirror and understand who I was and what I was running away from. Even as I am writing this book, I am being enlightened by the things that I like to do, navigating through my personal relationship with God, and making a more conscious decision to show up as my true authentic self. Therapy and Jesus have truly been helping me through this process. I have had to pull back the layers of my childhood, which shaped the woman I am today.

Seeking God's truth about who I am and who I should become has been challenging, as I have had to surrender many parts of my life to Him. Yet, I am reassured that all the things that I am seeking are falling into place. One of the things that I have realized is that perfection is relative and unrealistic for anyone to obtain in an imperfect world. I realized that I'd been living a lie, not a total lie, but a half-life. My self-awareness was nonexistent, and my self-perception was not accurate.

Although I am a giver by nature, I didn't realize just how selfish I was, nor did I realize how much of my identity was wrapped up in what society expected and what my parents and peers expected of me. I had to do a self-check and spend time in prayer daily so that I could hear God tell me who He wanted me to be. Upon further discovery, I noticed that I spent more time comparing myself to others than comparing myself to me. I also placed my identity and self-worth in my ability to be chosen by a man to be his wife and to have children. For a long time, this kept me back and had me living in fear and afraid that I'll never be married—afraid that God won't fulfill His promise to me.

It's amazing how you gain a different revelation when you read a Bible story over and over again. Recently, I read the story of Abraham and Sarah as they were waiting on the promise of a son in their very old age. Sarah decided she'd had enough waiting on God, so she took matters into her own hands. So, what did she do? She let her husband sleep with another woman—her servant—so that she could have a son. Back in those days, servants were property. If Sarah's servant bore a son by Abraham, that child would become Sarah's. At the time, it made logical sense. But those were not the instructions that God gave to Sarah.

Sarah looked at what was logical to fulfill the promise that God had made to her, but logic negates faith. God was testing Abraham and Sarah's faith. Although they made a whole mess of things, God still came through on His promise. I can't tell you the countless times when I allowed logic to negate my faith. Even on this journey to marriage and motherhood, I have meddled with God's truth over me time and time again. In these moments, I find that I have to silence the noise in my head, heart, and even my environment to get to the root of what may be causing doubt and my insecurities to override the voice of God. I have learned that the closer I draw nigh to God, the clearer things become and the less anxiety I feel.

Additionally, reading the Bible reminds me of His faithfulness. Not only that, reading my journal or diary of past prayers that were answered reminds me that God's got this, and God's got me. And He has you too! Never forget that the God who was faithful in the Bible is still faithful today. I am sure you can think of at least one time when your God has made good on His word to you. One thing I know for sure, God is not a man that He would lie to us. That is the Bible. Literally.

The reason why my self-perception had been off for so long was because my perception of God was off. I spent many years fearing God, which we should out of respect for Him. But many times, I found myself not trusting Him and only believing that He was a God of punishment and not the God of love that shows us grace and mercy daily. It wasn't until I began the journey of trusting God more that I truly began the journey of falling in love with myself. I had to fall in love with God to fall in love with myself.

Back in college is where I began to lose focus, and this is why this journey of self-awareness has been so important. My college sweetheart was a great guy, but I didn't know how to be in school and manage a relationship. I was more interested in dating and marrying him than I was in maintaining good grades. Believing I was in love, I gave him a precious gift—my virginity—because I was desperate to keep him in my life. Now that I'm older, I recognize that this is when I started displaying signs of having abandonment issues.

As a church girl, I was constantly torn between satisfying my flesh and not giving into temptation. I believe this is something many people struggle with, especially now that sex is thrown at us every day in the music we listen to, in what we watch, and on social media. The saying is "sex sells." Each time I gave into temptation, I felt incredibly guilty. It was as if I was unworthy of God's love.

I would cry all night long, repent, do well for a while, but then I would find myself back in the same predicament. Each time, I found myself making the conscious decision to sin and not flee from temptation like the Bible instructed me to do.[3] There must have been some sort of void that I found myself attempting to fill but was failing miserably at doing so. Just because I grew up in a loving home didn't mean I was immune to making poor choices in romantic partners. And these poor choices continued into my adulthood. For a while, I took a break from dating and found myself in quite a few "situationships," or relationships that I would be in for years but were never formal or established.

I spent years of my life trying to impress men who weren't ready to commit to me. My hope was always that the man I was with would see the light and lock me down, but that never happened. After years of this roller coaster ride and long periods of time not dating, I decided to officially get back in the dating game. Don't get me wrong, it wasn't that men didn't want me. There has always been the occasional DMer or creep who tried to get at me.

But usually, these guys weren't interesting to me, weren't my type, were thirsty, or just had way too much going on in their lives. For some reason, I attracted guys who needed healing or were way too broken for me to attempt to fix. I tried

---

[3] 1 Cor. 6:18 (NLT).

to improve some of them, but I couldn't. I grew to understand that I attracted the broken because I have the gift of healing; it all made sense after that. I moved on to online dating.

Since I didn't go to places outside of work and church to meet guys, I was sure I would meet someone online. At the suggestion of a matchmaker, I not only gave online dating a try, but I became a serial dater and dated multiple guys at once. My brother even went as far as to call me a player, but I corrected him and said I wasn't a player. It was just that I had a lot of options.

I explained to him that I wasn't a player because every guy I went on a date with knew that I was entertaining other men. Overall, my online dating experience was scary, overwhelming, ghetto, and unsuccessful. This was my "Sarah moment," and I sometimes blame myself because I was too afraid to try online dating when it first came out—before the creepers, sex offenders, prisoners (yes, prisoners), and desperate people took over the apps. I remember scrolling through my messages on one particular app one day and opening a message from a gentleman who seemed to be good looking.

After I started looking at his page, I began to see a pattern. Every photo he was in was taken in the same room but at a different angle, which wouldn't have been a huge red flag if the walls weren't all cinder blocks. My first thought was, *there is no way that this man is in jail, on a phone, and posting on this dating app.* Look, I know everybody needs love, but isn't a phone considered contraband in jail? I didn't even ask him whether he was in jail because the last photo in his gallery solidified my suspicions. He was wearing the blue-and-white-coordinated top and bottom that is common clothing for someone who is imprisoned. I immediately deleted our message thread without a second thought. I will say that I have dated a couple of men who were previously incarcerated but have turned their lives around and are doing very well now. However, I am not interested in dating men who are still in jail and using smuggled goods to reach out to me.

I tried free apps, Christian dating apps, paid apps, apps for professionals, and exclusive (waitlist) apps to no avail. All sorts of men reached out to me. Initially, I thought, *wow, there are so many options!* At one point, I even considered signing up for a dating service that cost over $2,000. As I pondered if the investment was worth it, I thought, *Am I really about to pay $2,000 just to date someone who could potentially NOT marry me?* I ended up not making the "investment" as the salesperson put it, but it got me thinking about what I really wanted in life.

I kept some messages on "read" and didn't respond to them for weeks, thinking I could give their senders a chance. When I did, I regretted taking the time to get to know many of the guys who were lucky enough to date me. Over time, I realized that many of these men were either desperate, lonely, or in need of some significant healing beyond my abilities. Honestly, you and I have had at least one cringeworthy relationship or situationship that we would like to forget, right?

You've run into the guy who is afraid of commitment, so he keeps you around—for years even—but never says, "Hey, let's be exclusive." Or we've dated the serial dater, the guy who lies about everything or the guy who has all the potential but none of the ambition. Let's not forget the guy with all the ambition but no potential because his arrogance is just so off-putting that we just can't. There is also the guy who shouldn't be dating because he is so broke that he is afraid that you are going to order more than water. Then, there is the guy who is perfect except for that one thing about his religion, his political affiliation, or his teeth (which, by the way, can be fixed). If none of the following describes any situationships you've been in, then one of three things has occurred:

1. You have been extremely blessed to date some amazing men.
2. You haven't really been dating.
3. You're a unicorn.

There really aren't any other explanations. However, if you're stuck on #2, let me help you a bit. Your man is not going to find you if you are not getting out of your house and making yourself seen. Additionally, please stop waiting for Boaz. Boaz was Ruth's man. Boaz was also married, Ruth's relative, and old. Now, if that's what you're looking for, then go ahead and be great, sis. But I hope that you're looking to marry someone who is not already married.

There are going to be some challenges, but you need to get out of the comfort of your own home, put on some real clothes, and meet men. Flirt a little. I know that rejection may be uncomfortable. You also may be trying to avoid the drama of a female cussing you out for approaching her man. But if you don't let it be known that you are available, men won't look your way twice. Don't be afraid to make eye contact or start a conversation. In a way, you need to be like Ruth and position yourself to be found. So, show a little leg.

Now look, I am not telling you to go out and show off all that God has given you that is appealing to men. Save that for the undefiled marriage bed. But if you want to catch a man's eye, you've got to give him something to look at. Your comfort level of showing off what your mama gave you may not be my comfort level. All I am saying is that wearing your holiness dress down to your ankles may not attract your husband to you. I would like for us to take a moment to let go of the notion that we have to be covered from our ear lobes to our ankles.

Let's admit it, this look is not only hot, but it's uncomfortable and outdated. There is a way to be sanctified and holy while still being comfortable and attractive. Now, you might be reading this and saying, how do I stay modest but show a little leg?

First, let's start with what you consider to be your best physical feature. It could be your arms, shoulders, or smile. For me, it is my legs and my derrière. When I am on a date, I may wear a midi skirt or a pencil skirt that is a little above the knee. I may also wear skinny jeans with a fitted shirt that is still sexy but tasteful. Second, let's get rid of the clothing items you've had since your teens that you either can't wear anymore or that never came back in style. Also, throw out that two-piece suit you wore to Convocation in the summer of 2001. I'll wait.

Yes, the one that you wore with the kitten heels and the white stockings. You know, the one with the butterfly collar? I am only joking, but it's always nice to stay contemporary. Watch the trends for your age group.

Third, wear clothes that fit you not just according to your size, but that also fit your personality. Wear clothes that bring out the best in you and make you feel confident. You don't have to break the bank to do this.

And like my mother told me, "Confidence is the new sexy." And men love confident women. Just stay relevant and appropriate for your body type. I will have to do a video on this because there is way too much to cover in this book. Also, feel free to contact me if you need help. I can help with styling, too. Just reach out to me at *www.allthingsalishaj.com*.

Whether you're showing a little leg or a bright smile (pair this with a fierce red lip, hunty), be confident in what you're wearing and show off your best asset! Another challenge I ran into was with guys who didn't respect my vow of celibacy.

During this period of my life, I was afraid that God would punish me if I didn't practice celibacy. Did I slip up and break my vow? Yes, I did quite a few times.

Dating in the 21st century is challenging when dealing with men who have been exposed to sex since they were children. There is also the hurdle that men typically are not the ones who are encouraged to remain virgins until marriage. I found that, in being in a committed relationship, it was normal for sex to be expected. To clarify, not all the men I dated had this mindset. Some men respected my decision to remain celibate, but they were few.

I want to take this time to express that cold showers don't work. Have you been turned on by a date or two and tried to take a cold shower thinking it was going help cool things down? Did that work for you? Because it surely did not work for me. I mean, all I ended up feeling was more frustrated than I was before I got into the shower. If that works for you, keep doing you, sis. But I am going to share three things I did to help remain celibate and avoid temptation:

1. Pray.
2. Keep men out of my house and keep my butt out of theirs.

3. Wear spanks.

To my first point, the first line of defense is always prayer. Truth moment. I have gone on dates where I was so intensely attracted to the man, I was dating that my vagina marched to the beat of her own drum. Can you relate? I remember times when I have cried because I was so sexually frustrated and would ask God why I couldn't just do the deed so that I did not have to suffer. Sis, this road has been rough. You hear me?

If you are a virgin, please remain one. Once that door has been opened, it's hard to close. Just keep that door locked and throw away the key until you're married. The amount of discipline it takes to keep yourself from falling into sin after you know what it feels like to have sex is more difficult than it was when you only imagined what the deed was like. Plus, soul ties take time to get healed and delivered from. Just don't do it, sis. One time, when I was at the house of a man I was dating, I actually started humming the children's Sunday school favorite "Jesus Loves Me, This I Know" just to avoid going too far. He stopped kissing me. Staring into my eyes, he asked, "Are you humming 'Jesus Loves Me, This I Know?"

I told him I was, and we got a good laugh out of it. He was one of the good guys I dated, but we could never get it together. I learned a lot from that relationship. Don't settle for someone who isn't fully ready to be with you. If you are dedicated to being completely celibate, don't settle with a man who just can't handle it. If he decides that your decision is too much to handle, let him walk away. Trust me, there are men that will respect your choice and make adjustments to ensure you keep your promise to God. In my times of struggle, I remember praying this distinct prayer: "Dear Lord, my vagina and my body want to have sex. I am extremely attracted to this man, and I am doing the best that I can to remain holy because I want to please you. Please help a sister out and keep me from sinning. In Jesus' name, Amen."

I ain't gonna lie to y'all (I am purposefully saying it like this because I need you to hear me), my prayer did not always work. Why? Because my heart was not always in the right place.

There were times I prayed this prayer or a similar prayer. I had my heart set on fulfilling my own selfish desires, so I did what I was tempted to do or what I wanted to do. You were probably hoping that the prayer would solve all your problems, but God gives us free will. So, unless we're willing to make a change, nothing will change.

If your mind is in the place to give into temptation and sin, then that is what you will do. But if you really want to overcome sin and still date, then I suggest you refer to suggestion number two. Don't go to his house and don't have him spend the night at yours. You may think, *well, I won't have any issues in this area because it's been so long since I've done something, so a little cuddling won't hurt.* You're right, a little cuddling won't hurt. But a little cuddling becomes a lot of cuddling, then a little petting, and so on and so forth. Before you know it, you're back at the altar on Sunday morning asking God for forgiveness.

It's literally common sense. Don't set yourself up for failure and you won't fail. Trust me, I know from experience. A guy I started dating spent the night twice. We did not have sex, but it was very difficult not to. After the second time we stayed together, he told me that he couldn't spend the night anymore. It was too much for him. To my surprise, he didn't give me an ultimatum, but he made it clear that he and I could not be alone together at each other's houses, no matter how much we liked cuddling with each other. And I am a CUDDLER.

So, my first reaction was "why?!" (Cue dramatic tears here.) This has never happened before, where a man was mature enough to tell me that he couldn't handle it but still wanted to see me.

He didn't reject me or stop talking to me. He just shifted how we dated. I shared this story so that you understand that there are guys who will respect your wishes. They may not be mature enough to initiate the conversation, but they are out there. Don't doubt God. Your husband will find you.

Third, if at first you don't succeed, dust yourself off and try some spanks or a good body shaper. You know, the ones with the shorts that you literally have to jump into and run out of breath putting on. I'm not talking about the ones that are crotchless either (that defeats the whole point). I know it sounds crazy, but if you wrestle against fat and bulge, you know the struggle it takes to put on spanks. So, another practical way to avoid falling into sin is to wrap yourself up in garments that are not easy to get out of. It takes about as much effort to take those bad boys off, too. Now, I know this may not work all the time (because who wants to wear spanks to a date at a baseball game), but it is definitely an option that works.

You may be thinking, *why didn't she say anything about an accountability partner?* Let's be honest, if you are in the moment and have it in your mind that you are going to do the deed, no number of friends calling or texting to check on you is going to stop you. In fact, you will probably ignore your phone at that point. Not to mention, as much as we love our friends or family members, they can let us down as well.

They may fall asleep, like John, Peter, and James when Jesus asked them to watch and pray right before He was to be arrested to go to the cross.[4] Or they may forget to be praying for your strength in the Lord. Trust me, it happens (especially if you're on a date until the wee hours of the morning). I will add a disclaimer. Some of us have friends that have been real ones since day one, and they will pull up at your house (or his house, if you gave them the address) to make sure you don't fall. These types of friends are rare, but they do exist.

Although challenging, celibacy is possible. You just have to be disciplined and prayerful. Despite the responses I get now, I am even more committed to celibacy because I love God and don't want to disappoint Him. Now, in moments

---

[4] Mark 14: 32 – 52 (NLT).

of temptation, it is easier to say "no" to a relationship where sex is expected and walk away because my "why" has changed.

I have gone from having a mindset of condemnation to one of a longing to please God. While on the dating apps, I also began to take marriage prep classes. I read books about wholeness, and I joined dating boot camps and challenges that coached me through praying for my spouse. But it didn't stop there.

I attended courses to learn how to be a wife, did speed dating, and even put in an application to be on a dating show. I tried to prepare to be a wife and threw my Hail Mary to no avail. The overachiever in me had difficulty tying down a man, so I began to question my worthiness and compatibility altogether. As I wrestled with my inability to land a man, I also began to ask God if I would ever get married. He'd spoken through several prophets that I would be married and give birth.

So, I finally got to the point where I asked Him what He was doing because I didn't see a husband anywhere in sight. This was when I realized it was because I had made being married and becoming a mother my gods. These two things consumed my life. I was more concerned with becoming what the world deemed "blessed" than becoming who God called me to be. He reminded me of a verse in the Bible that says, "An unmarried woman or virgin is concerned about the Lord's affairs: Her aim is to be devoted to the Lord in both body and spirit."[5]

I'd lost all focus of where my devotion was, so I had to repent and return to becoming the woman God had called me to be. In the back of my mind, I thought a man would not want to date me because of the infertility diagnosis I had received. I feared that sharing my fertility status with whomever I dated would discourage him from wanting to continue pursuing me or even consider marrying me. But I found that most of the men I dated either already had kids and didn't want more, were open to adoption, or had more faith than I did that I would give birth.

When we are in our unmarried season, it is important for us to remember that it is just that, a season, and the season will not last forever. "When are you going to get married?" "When are you going to have children?" These are two questions that I hate to have to answer. As a society, we have to do better at starting conversations this way.

---

[5] 1 Cor. 7:34 (NIV).

These two questions are triggers for so many, and for women who aren't dating, these questions are almost impossible to answer. A really close friend of mine suggested that we respond with "did you brush your teeth this morning?" I laughed because this response was so hilarious! But it's such an awesome response. I mean, think about it. She was just matching energy to energy. The question posed was personal, so the response, although a question, is equally as intrusive.

Church girls can also get spooky or spiritual with it and respond with an arbitrary time because we are "naming it and claiming it." But the Bible states that we have not because our motives are wrong.[6] What if that is not what God has planned for you next week? Next month? Next year? Yes, God knows you desire to be married.

He knew that before you were born. He knows how old you are right now, and He knows what your reproductive organs are doing as well. It is not our responsibility to know the who, what, where, when, how, and why. We are responsible for putting our faith to work and walking in our purpose while we wait. So, the next time you're asked about

---

[6] James 4:3 (NLT).

when you will get married or have children, respond by saying, "God is writing my love story, but while I wait, I am walking in my purpose and living by faith."

God wants our focus to be on Him and what He has purposed us to do. After I stopped chasing marriage and motherhood, I began to focus on my life. I became a preacher, bought a house, and paid more attention to helping others. I confessed to some of the men that I liked them, then left the ball in their courts. One guy that I confessed to asked me to give him more time. I told him I couldn't promise that because I was over waiting for him to make up his mind and I knew my worth.

I reminded myself daily that I am the prize. I am the good thing. He who finds me finds favor with the Lord. I became more intentional about spending more time with my Abba. I embraced my "rich aunty season," a time to focus on building my wealth, traveling, and living my best life. I realized I had the freedom to move how I wanted within God's plans. After I surrendered my desires, many other doors began to open for me. Things continue to unfold even as I write this book. God is good!

My prayer for you:

Abba, please keep my sister from all counterfeits. May she not encounter men who have ill intentions. I ask that you please send her a man who loves You, who has integrity, and has good character. We also ask that he has good credit, is attractive to her, and is submitted to You, so that she can submit to him, and they can submit to one another (Eph. 5: 21 – 64).

Abba, I ask that You give my sister courage, and may she be confident that she will see Your goodness manifested in her life as she puts herself out there to date (Ps. 27: 13 – 14).

As she is waiting and dating, may she be devoted to You and holy in body and in spirit so that she can serve You whole heartedly without distractions (1 Cor. 7:34).

I pray that she desires to please you with her body and that she and her fiancé remains celibate until their honeymoon night (I Cor. 6:18-19) and that she and her husband will fully enjoy married sex (Heb. 13:4).

I ask that she will be confident in knowing that her love story will be more beautiful than she could ever imagine because You are the author (Heb. 12:2).

Please grant her the desires of her heart (Ps. 37:4) and may she glorify You when Your promises are fulfilled in her life. In Jesus' name I pray this prayer. Amen.

Chapter 3
The Diagnosis

"For I know the plans I have for you," says the Lord. "They are plans for good and not for disaster, to give you a future and a hope."

–Jeremiah 29:11 (NLT)

How did I get here? Remember when I mentioned that I typically got hot flashes during my cycle? Well, I originally thought nothing of it whenever I got them. I recall one study session in college when I had a flash so severe that I cranked the window unit air conditioner in my sophomore dorm to the max and more than likely froze my study buddies to the bone.

I thought nothing of it though, even years to follow. I would occasionally ask my OB-GYN about having hot flashes during my cycle and every time I'd ask, regardless of my doctor's race or gender, I was told that this was normal.

However, in 2018, my hot flashes began to intensify, which made me believe something in my body was off. As time progressed, I began to get night sweats as well. I was incredibly moody and irritable while experiencing fibroids and ovarian cysts, which I'd had since high school.

The fibroids caused me to bleed heavily for weeks on end, causing a great deal of inconvenience. Namely, I made a lot of investment in sanitary napkins, had discomfort sitting in blood for weeks, and experienced leaks (no matter how "super" the pad was). I remember doubling up on panties to make sure the pad didn't move during the night, only to find that whatever position I laid in the night before proved to be unsuccessful because the sheets bore my blood stains in the morning. Not to mention, my right ovary was a great source of pain. It became so intense that I had to go to the hospital.

My first experience at the hospital to address ovarian pain was memorable but not in a good way. It was around the time when I was launching my first ministry called Church Girl DNA, a non-profit organization that was created to encourage and empower all church girls regardless of age. As I sat in the hospital with my mother, the nurse seemed annoyed when she told me that they were having difficulty locating my right ovary, but I felt what I felt. I was in excruciating pain to the point of tears.

I thought my right ovary was dying for sure, but as she continued to probe, the pain I felt was no longer just in my ovaries. I sat on the hospital bed and tried to convince the medical professional that I wasn't lying about the pain I was feeling. I felt unheard and disregarded. The nurse was a white woman. I am not sure if she was being discriminatory, but it felt like she was at that moment.

I left the ER with a hefty bill. Still in pain, I got no solution that night. But my mother got a chance to minister and pray for a church member down the hall. The pain I was feeling kept me in bed, and I almost canceled the launch of my ministry. But I pressed on, and Church Girl DNA launched. My ministry has since evolved into All Things Alisha J. as I have lumped all the things I do under one umbrella, including empowering women, running a clothing boutique, doing speaking services, providing infertility support, and so many other things.

I wish the nurse had listened to me when I was in the hospital because a cyst burst in my right ovary later, and I thought I was going to meet my Maker. The first time I experienced a cyst bursting was as I was driving on my way to work one morning. If you haven't experienced this, it feels like an explosion has occurred in your ovary and is followed by a pulse of constant pain. I couldn't move. I was paralyzed by the pain, and I thought I was going to have to pull the car over because I wanted to curl up into a ball. The pain subsided after a few minutes, and I was able to make it to work safely.

Years later, I experienced the same thing a second time. I was in the shower, and I felt my body get hot. Then, an overwhelming feeling came over me. Then the pain hit, again, in the same right ovary. It felt as though my whole reproductive system was about to fall out of my body. I was on my cycle at the time and was in so much pain that I called my parents. Living alone at the time, I was afraid I was dying.

I'd just surpassed the age that my biological mother was when she died from leukemia. Fear gripped me and I couldn't help but think that God was calling me home to be with Him and my mother. I wasn't ready to leave, so I needed some help. My dad answered the phone, and he began to get more uneasy as he heard the panic in my voice. My supernatural mother was nearby and could hear both of us, so she provided the calm we both needed.

She called one of my aunties who lived nearby and asked her to come and see about me. She also called the ambulance. In retrospect, I should have asked her not to, but I was afraid for my life. Ambulance rides are expensive. I lived less than a few miles from the nearest hospital, so it was a waste. When my auntie got to my house, I didn't think I was going to make it to the door to open it. I believe she and the paramedics arrived around the same time.

I crawled from the bedroom to the door, then I crawled to the bathroom to put on a house dress. I had not brushed my teeth at this point and was so embarrassed by my appearance because, to my surprise, all three of the EMT workers were good looking gentlemen. They asked some very probing questions about whether I was pregnant, and I told one of them several times that I was celibate. I understood that his line of questioning could have been to help determine how to better assist me, but I got annoyed at the lead paramedic because he was being very pushy. I was also embarrassed because, although I was in pain, I was aware of the fact that I did not look my best. I thought to myself, *of all days, when I don't look all the way together and my breath stinks, God, you send three handsome men to my door.* The irony.

They loaded me up on the gurney and into the ambulance. Once I got into the ambulance, I was no longer in pain. I was too embarrassed to say anything about no longer being in pain, but I wish I had as it would have saved me some money. But hindsight is 20/20, right? So, there I was in the ambulance alone with a house dress and nothing to catch my flow. I was embarrassed on so many levels, but I can now say that I have ridden in an ambulance once in my life and plan on never doing so again.

My parents met me in the emergency room and were such a great support system. The doctors and nurses were so much friendlier than my previous experience with the nurse who didn't believe me years earlier. This was actually the first time someone explained to me that it was possibly an ovarian cyst and that I would be fine. I did some research and found out that ovarian cysts are fluid-filled sacs or pockets in an ovary or on its surface. It is common for women to have ovarian cysts at some time, and many don't even know they have them because the cysts don't cause them any pain or discomfort.

Fortunately, most ovarian cysts are harmless and disappear without treatment within a few months.[7] Studying further, I also learned that uterine fibroids may appear as noncancerous growths of the uterus during childbearing years. They can range in size and may be as small as a seed, which can be undetectable to the human eye, or as large as a mass that can enlarge the uterus. You can have multiple fibroids at once, and sometimes fibroids can even cause weight gain.[8] After my trip to the ER, I felt educated and empowered about the condition of my ovaries. I then followed up with my primary care provider (PCP) and obstetrician-gynecologist (OB-GYN), who had been monitoring the health of my ovaries and my reproductive system.

I still have ovarian cysts, but they haven't been nearly as dramatic lately. During my follow-up with my doctor, I had additional tests done. My PCP took a series of blood tests to assess my levels. I told her about the hot flashes and night sweats, which prompted her to check my thyroid and anti-

---

[7] "Ovarian Cysts - Symptoms and Causes," Mayo Clinic, August 6, 2022, https://www.mayoclinic.org/diseases-conditions/ovarian-cysts/symptoms-causes/syc-20353405.

[8] Mayo Clinic. "Uterine Fibroids - Symptoms and Causes," September 21, 2022. https://www.mayoclinic.org/diseases-conditions/uterine-fibroids/symptoms-causes/syc-20354288.

Müllerian hormone (AMH) levels to see if I was going through early onset menopause. Typically, AMH levels for fertile women are between 1.0–4.0 nanograms per milliliter (ng/ml). Less than 1.0 ng/ml is considered low and indicates a diminished ovarian reserve.

When my tests came back, my AMH levels were 0.03 ng/ml. Yes, you read that correctly. At 0.03 ng/mL, my egg reserve was pretty much nonexistent, and my chances of getting pregnant, according to science, was slim to none.[9] My PCP also measured my follicle-stimulating hormone (FSH) levels. FSH is a hormone associated with reproduction and the development of eggs in women. The pituitary gland, a small organ located in the center of the head behind the sinus cavity at the base of the brain, makes FSH.

Among my age group, a normal FSH level is between 4.7 to 21.5 milli-international units per milliliter (mIU/mL). A typical range for women going through menopause is between 25.8 to 134.8 mIU/mL.[10]

---

[9] "Anti-Müllerian Hormone Test," n.d. https://medlineplus.gov/lab-tests/anti-mullerian-hormone-test/.

[10] Goldberg, Joanna. "Follicle-Stimulating Hormone (FSH) Test." Healthline, September 17, 2018. https://www.healthline.com/health/fsh.

My levels came back at around 110 mIU/mL, which meant that I was considered perimenopausal and, according to my doctors, experiencing pre-ovarian failure.[11] After receiving word from my PCP that my thyroid test was as expected but the other tests came back abnormal, she suggested I go to my OB-GYN right away to get a second opinion. Well, I dragged my feet to make the appointment with my OB-GYN, but I finally did it.

A few days after my appointment, my doctor called me to deliver my results. I recall the sadness in her voice as she told me about my devastatingly abnormal AMH and FSH levels. She explained that I was either experiencing pre-ovarian failure or I was in the beginning stages of perimenopause (transitioning to becoming menopausal). After hearing the news, I think I stopped breathing. My life flashed before my eyes. I thought, *Menopause at thirty-four? Like, who does that?*

After hanging up the call with my OB-GYN, I called my best friend and ugly cried. For the first time in my life, my faith was tested in an area I never thought I'd have difficulty in,

---

[11] Follicle-Stimulating Hormone (FSH) Levels Test," n.d. https://medlineplus.gov/lab-tests/follicle-stimulating-hormone-fsh-levels-test/.

especially being unmarried. That day, I was introduced to a word that was not in my vocabulary: infertility. I thought, *what is this? What is this God-ordained season I am entering?*

My best friend, who was pregnant with my godson, cried with me and paid attention to my needs even though she was on vacation with her husband. I was a bit hesitant to call her because I'd been advised to be cognizant of the stress that this would cause her and how that could potentially drive her into premature labor. But I needed someone to talk to and a shoulder to lean on. I was devastated. I cried to the point of screaming. I sat alone in my apartment with my tears and my feelings.

I called my parents as well and cried. I was just so hurt. I remember wondering, *how could a merciful and loving God call my natural mother to be home with Him and then take my ability to become a mother away from me?* Back then, I just couldn't grasp what was going on with what I considered to be a difficult time landing a husband and being a late bloomer. It hit me like a ton of bricks that my journey to marriage was challenging, but now my journey to motherhood would even be more challenging.

I am a mover and a shaker, so I didn't stay in this head space for long before I started exploring my options.

According to the Centers for Disease Control and Prevention (CDC), infertility is defined as not being able to get pregnant after trying for one year.[12] Factors contributing to infertility may include uterine fibroids, weight gain, trauma, stress, and more. According to Resolve, black women are 1.5 times more likely to experience infertility than women of other races.[13]

I mention this because I am blessed that both of my doctors are black Christian females who pay closer attention to my needs as a black woman when it comes to my health.

In a world where black women are mishandled when it comes to fertility and childbirth, it is important that you select a team of physicians that can relate and care for you in a way that is beneficial to your health both mentally and emotionally.[14] Perhaps infertility doesn't exactly describe what I am going through because I haven't been

---

[12] "Infertility | Reproductive Health | CDC," n.d. https://www.cdc.gov/reproductivehealth/infertility/index.htm.

[13] RESOLVE: The National Infertility Association. "KTC: Sharing Our Story - A Conversation About Infertility in the Black Community." Video. *YouTube*, March 5, 2021. https://www.youtube.com/watch?v=y0bf8GBml6k.

[14] RESOLVE: The National Infertility Association, "KTC: Sharing Our Story - A Conversation About Infertility in the Black Community."

actively trying to get pregnant, so I will consider myself as " fertility challenged." Maybe, I'll make this a catch phrase.

Regardless, there definitely needs to be more awareness brought to fertility challenges in the African American community. Thus, the reason I am writing this book.

I want you, the reader, to be more aware of your reproductive ability, so you can make more informed choices when you begin your journey to motherhood. After calling and crying with my family and friends, I took the next step to discuss my options with my doctors. My OB-GYN referred me to a reproduction specialist, and I started the process of freezing my eggs. My consultation with the specialist was an eye-opener because he informed me that I was not alone. He shared with me that, over his twenty-five-year career, he'd encountered teenage girls who were also perimenopausal.

He further explained that my chances of having eggs to retrieve were slim to none, but he would try anyway. Getting your eggs frozen is not cheap. This process was not covered by insurance and so I had to come up with almost $12,000 to freeze my eggs. Then, there is an additional cost to store the eggs in a special freezer, retrieve them from the freezer, perform in vitro fertilization (IVF), and attend follow up doctor's visits. During this time, I'd lost my high-salaried job and was living off severance pay.

Even with financial challenges, I was determined to do what I could to become a mother. As always, my faithful Abba provided the funds I needed to start the process of freezing my eggs. Before I could begin freezing my eggs, there were a million consent forms to fill out and several different blood tests performed to ensure I was a qualified candidate for the process. Many of my appointments included having ultrasounds and tracking my cycles, which were so inconsistent that it became challenging to begin hormone therapy. After a few months of waiting for my first cycle, I finally began the first step of follicle aspiration, or egg retrieval. To get to the eggs, you have to retrieve the follicle, a small, fluid-filled sac in the ovary that contains one immature egg.

When an egg matures during a woman's menstrual cycle, the follicle breaks open and releases the egg from the ovary for possible fertilization (the process by which an egg combines with sperm to form an embryo).[15] Basically, this was done to trick my body into producing more than one follicle to do the extraction. I had to inject hormones into my stomach four times a day like clockwork, which was not fun. The needles were small, but it was still painful because I had to inject them in my stomach. Finding different injection sites every day became really tricky. Also, all the vials of hormones had to be kept refrigerated.

    The week that I had to inject myself was during a time when I was unemployed. It was convenient for me to keep up with my injection schedule since I could do it from the comfort of my own home. Although invasive and unbelievable, I still believed. I had everybody and their mamas praying that my levels would miraculously increase so that the specialist could retrieve at least ten follicles with at least ten good eggs that could be frozen. I would go into the prayer room of my apartment and pray fervently for two things: a husband and ten follicles with eggs.

---

[15] IVI, "What Is a Follicle and How Many Follicles Do You Need?", IVI Fertility, April 12, 2022, https://ivi-fertility.com/blog/follicle-how-many-follicles-do-you-need/.

I still believe, although my prayers have changed slightly. After my last shot, I headed to the specialist to get the ultrasound that would reveal how many follicles were available for the egg retrieval. My appointment was on a Sunday because my last shot and the ultrasound had to be synched. I remember lying on the table in the room alone and praying for a change. Just like the nurse in the ER several years before, the ultrasound tech initially had a hard time finding my right ovary.

I recall the look on her face as she tried to locate my ovaries. I perceived that she had not found any follicles and I sensed that she wanted to tell me the news herself, but she was unable to tell me the results. She was very pleasant and personable as she instructed me to clean up and redress. She then proceeded to let me know that the nurse would more than likely contact me once they received the results. I thanked her, left the facility, and headed to church.

All the while, I still prayed for a miracle. During church service, I saw my phone's indicator light flashing. I had received a missed call from the reproductive clinic. I stepped out of the sanctuary and hid in one of the offices to return the call. The nurse on the other end told me, "Ms. Blanding, there were no follicles found. I am so sorry, but we have to cancel your cycle." I will never forget those words. After I hung up the phone, I sat in the office and cried.

The word "cancel" rang in my head. When I returned to the sanctuary, I tried my best to hold back the tears, but it seemed as though they fell harder the more, I fought them back. Eventually, I made eye contact with my mama in the pulpit. I could tell she knew something was wrong. After service, I went to the altar and wept. I suppose it was similar to the way Hannah wept when she asked God for a son.[16] The word "cancel" changed my life. It stung, but it also gave me a purpose.

My prayer for you:

Abba, I pray that my dear sister accepts your timeline for her life and that she trusts that You will grant her the patience she needs as she waits for Your promises to manifest (II Cor. 1:20).

I pray that as she seeks You for direction, that she will find the answers that she is looking for and that because we know You to be a good Abba, we know that You will

---

[16] 1 Sam. 1 (NLT).

give her good gifts if she asks for them You (Matt. 7:7 – 8).

I am believing with my sister that no good thing will You keep from her (Ps. 84:11) and that You will bless her womb to carry children to full term just like you blessed the wombs of Sarah, Hannah, Elizabeth, and so many other women in the Bible.

In faith we believe you to be Jehovah Rophe, our healer and we stand in agreement that You will heal and provide. In Jesus' name I pray this prayer. Amen.

Chapter 4
The Blame Game

So now there is no condemnation for those who belong to Christ Jesus. And because you belong to him, the power of the life-giving Spirit has freed you from the power of sin that leads to death. The law of Moses was unable to save us because of the weakness of our sinful nature. So, God did what the law could not do. He sent his own Son in a body like the bodies we sinners have. And in that body God declared an end to sin's control over us by giving his Son as a sacrifice for our sins. He did this so that the just requirement of the law would be fully satisfied for us, who no longer follow our sinful nature but instead follow the Spirit.

–Romans 8:1 -4 (NLT)

As a child, my summers were filled with exploration, curiosity, and love. I remember baking cakes with my grandmother and getting eggs with her from the chicken coop. I was blessed because my parents grew up less than twenty minutes away from each other. Each summer, I rotated between my father's side of the family and my mother's side. I recall running up and down dirt roads where I spent time learning how to double Dutch, playing jacks, and draw box outlines for hopscotch.

The smell of the rain in the Lowcountry and the loud sound it made as the water bounced off the tin roof enticed me to go back to a simpler time in life. Sometimes, my cousins and I sat on the porch during rainy days and helped my grandmother shuck peas as we were eaten alive by mosquitos. Back in those days, there wasn't a care in the world. There was freedom. There was life. There was innocence . . . until there wasn't.

One summer proved to be the catalyst for why I go to therapy today. The majority of my cousins and I are around the same age, so we customarily played together outside when we were younger (this was so the grown folks had time to themselves). Like most children, we "played house" and pretended to be husband and wife. We'd played this game many times before without any issues. I was the wife, and he was the husband. It was good, clean fun until he decided to take his role as husband beyond child's play.

The first time it happened, I knew something was off. I thought, *this doesn't seem right, but I don't know what doesn't seem right. I don't like how this feels, but I am going along with it because we are playing house.* As I reflect on what happened now as an adult, I realize that he must have been regularly exposed to what he was doing to me because he knew exactly what to do. He stole from me something that was stolen from him.

It was almost like he purposely pursued me, every time we were alone, to do the things that only married, consenting adults should do. Eventually, I no longer enjoyed playtime with my cousin and began to hate being around him. One day, I found myself alone with him on the porch. Helpless, I lay there, once again, not enjoying what was being done to me. No more than a few seconds later, someone approached.

I thought they were coming to rescue me, but I was wrong. It all happened so quickly. The family member came storming out on the porch and began to whoop me and my cousin. Not only was I violated, but I was also punished for being violated. I didn't want to be there. But I was there, and I felt even more abandoned than before. As an adult, I understand that my family member did what they thought was best.

They were trying to ensure that my cousin and I wouldn't do anything unholy ever by beating us. When I was around nine years old, my supernatural mother asked me if I wanted to stop going to South Carolina in the summer. It was like the Holy Spirit told her that something had happened to me and that I no longer needed to go there. As a nine-year-old, it was difficult for me to tell her why I no longer wanted to go because I wasn't sure if what happened was good or bad.

I told my mom that I no longer wanted to go to South Carolina, and that was that. I began this chapter talking about the things that caused me physical, emotional, and mental pain because these memories were brought back to my mind. Along the way, I convinced myself that the encounters with my cousin contributed to me being diagnosed with infertility. I believed the root of my addiction to porn and the loss of my virginity were tied to the molestation I experienced as a child. In my mind, God was punishing me for being violated, just like I'd been punished as a child.

Looking back, I see that the enemy used these situations to keep me bound. When I received the infertility diagnosis, I considered every minor infraction that I committed against God as His reason for keeping me from being married and able to conceive. My mind raced with a million what-if thoughts. *What if I hadn't allowed my cousin to violate me? What if I had never become addicted to porn? What if I hadn't lost my virginity? What if I had truly committed myself to being celibate instead of giving in to temptation?*

I lived in guilt for years after losing my virginity in college. When I returned to my parent's' home the summer after it happened, I remember the guilt literally eating me alive. I lived in it. Every time my mother mentioned how proud she was of me for remaining a virgin, I laughed and lied to her face. But I had to maintain my Perfect Patty persona. I had to keep up the façade and make my parents proud.

Because of the guilt, I overcompensated by being overly nice to my brother, who was more of an enemy than a friend at the time. I was overly helpful. My hope was that my actions would redeem me from my sins, but the only redemption for sin comes through repentance. I was not only fornicating, but I was lying about it to myself, my parents, and even God. I was stressing myself out trying to hide my sin, like Adam and

Eve in the Garden. But like the Bible says, any and everything that is done in the dark, will come to the light.[17]

A spotlight hit my sin on a day that was normal, so everything came to light. My body physically carried the weight of my sins to the point that I felt burdened 24/7. One day, my mother and I had a girl chat in the great room, the room your eyes first land on when you enter through the foyer of the house. The intricacy of the decorations of this room could not beautify the dirtiness of my sin and shame. As we spoke, my mother proceeded to talk about purity and remaining a virgin. We were specifically talking about some friends of mine and how they were no longer virgins.

Again, my mother was beaming with pride as she looked at me, thinking that her daughter was still a flower that had not been plucked. I can remember thinking, *God, please don't let her ask me if I am still a virgin*, because I knew I wasn't going to be able to lie. God must have known that I needed to release myself from the shame because the look on my face when she asked told on me before I could confirm the answer with my mouth. My mother's reaction was one of disappointment.

---

[17] Luke 12:2-3 (NIV).

We didn't talk for a few days. She still loved me and cared for me because, at the end of the day, I am still her child. I know it was hard for her to hear and comprehend, and I understand where she was coming from more now than when I was in my twenties.

As time went on, the weight of my guilt and shame lifted. I began living in my truth, and the relationship between my mother and I went back to normal. I am not sure how long it took to get there, but I am sure my mother had to forgive me and move on, even without getting a formal apology from me. I also went back to antagonizing my brother because I no longer felt the need to overcompensate for the guilt.

But the struggle was still real. I wrestled between pleasing my flesh or pleasing God. I failed. I failed God. *Because I failed*, I thought, *God is punishing me. He is keeping me from attaining everything I'd hoped for, prayed for, and ever wanted*. I didn't realize that I was making up a narrative that wasn't true.

Romans 8:1 says, "There is therefore now no condemnation to them which are in Christ Jesus, who walk not after the flesh, but after the Spirit" (KJV). At the time, I wasn't living in the freedom that God had called me to live in. I wasn't taking advantage of His grace, kindness, and favor toward me. God is a redeeming God. He is a loving God. And most importantly, He is a forgiving God.

God has forgiven me time and time again. So, my infertility diagnosis wasn't a punishment for anything that I'd done. It was just a part of my story—a portion of the testimony of what God can and will do for me and others. I realized that God trusted me enough to carry this because He knew I would use it to help, educate, and free others from pain, guilt, and shame. He knew He could trust me to give Him the glory throughout the process, even with my pity parties.

Now, I view it as an honor to be in the position I'm in. If you are wondering why God has chosen you to be unmarried or diagnosed with some form of fertility challenge, it is not because of anything you have done or didn't do. God is *not* punishing you. He is adding to your story to build your faith. I know this sounds easier said than done, but today, forgive yourself just as God has forgiven you. I want to encourage you to stop blaming yourself for something that God has ordained. You are *not* cursed. You are *not* broken. God is *not* done with you yet.

My prayer for you:

Abba, there has been something in all our lives that has shaped us to be the women we are today. I pray that my dear sister will not blame herself for whatever trauma or violation that occurred to her.

May she know that You have never and will never leave her nor forsake her (Deut. 31:8) and that all things work together for her good because she loves You (Rom. 8:28).

May she break up with thoughts of unworthiness and fear, for you have not given us a spirt of fear but one of love, power, and a sound mind (II Tim. 1:7).

I pray that she remembers that she is not condemned (Rom. 8:1) and that she has the power to cast down all imaginations that come against the knowledge of You and subject them to the power of Jesus Christ (II Cor. 10:5).

I pray that she rests in the fact that You love her beyond what she could ask, think or imagine (Eph. 3:20) and that Your banner over her is love (Songs of Songs 2:4). In Jesus' name I pray this prayer. Amen

Chapter 5
The Seven Stages of Grief

You keep track of all my sorrows. You have collected all my tears in your bottle. You have recorded each one in your book.

–Psalm 56:8 (NLT)

Who died? I don't know about you, but when I was initially diagnosed with infertility, my dream of becoming a mother and having a nuclear family died. It's not really a who but rather a what died. The idea of having kids slowly disappeared. There was a season when I grieved for the hopes and dreams, I had for my life before I accepted reality for what it was. My grieving period included many nights filled with tears. I yelled. I screamed. I questioned God's almighty power.

It was especially difficult to accept my reality on days when I received text messages announcing a pregnancy or engagement. I asked God when my turn would come. Was He trying to torture me? Although I was happy for my friend or family member, I felt sad for myself. It never really got easier until I realized that I needed to properly grieve the death of my dreams. Notice, I didn't say the death of my *womb* but the death of the way *I* thought things should be.

So, what is grief? It is what we experience mentally when we suffer an affliction or loss. In other words, it is painful sorrow or regret. There are seven commonly known stages of grief: shock and denial, pain and guilt, anger and bargaining, depression, upward turn, reconstruction and working through, and acceptance and hope.[18]

Stage 1: Shock & Denial

When I heard the news about being infertile, I was totally in shock. The announcement that I would not become a mother in the traditional way was a sudden and violent blow to my emotions and ego. I can be a proud person, and like I stated before, I had a perfect image of what my life would

---

[18] "7 Stages of Grief - Going through the Process and Back to Life," Recover From Grief, October 20, 2020, http://www.recover-from-grief.com/7-stages-of-grief.html.

look like. I was already behind on my timeline to be married. According to my calculations, I was supposed to be married at twenty-five, have my first kid around twenty-seven, and birth twins by thirty.

You see, I had everything all figured out, but God had a different plan for my life. And the day I found out that my chances of getting pregnant naturally were slim to none, it was like He threw a monkey wrench into Perfect Patty's world. Nothing made sense to me. I didn't understand how a pastor's kid, faithful servant, praise team leader, dance team member, intercessor, wise friend, and leader could be afflicted with the obstacles I faced. Was I not worthy enough to be blessed like the Bible said? **Proverbs 31:28 says, "Her children rise up and call her blessed" (AMP).** In Luke 23:29, it says, **"For the days are coming when they will say, 'Fortunate indeed are the women who are childless, the wombs that have not borne a child and the breasts that have never nursed'" (NLT).**

All my life I thought that only women who bore children were blessed, but even God had a scripture for those considered barren. Although comforting to know, the passage in Luke refers to a not-so-pleasant time for humanity as a whole (but this is not a theology book). I remember feeling shocked on the first Mother's Day after receiving the diagnosis. I cried all day at church. Then, I cried when I got home and tried to sleep the whole day away.

My heart was in pain. My body was in pain. My soul was hurting. I was in total shock all over again. It snuck up on me like a ninja. I thought I was fine, but no, there was a major reminder that the thing I cherished would be almost impossible to accomplish on my own. Remember, I said "on my own."

Then, after the shock came the denial. I remember telling myself that nothing was real. The doctors got it wrong. Maybe there were more follicles they didn't see because they had such a hard time locating my right ovary. Maybe my faith wasn't strong enough and that's why they didn't see the follicles. Then, I got to the point where reality had to meet my faith. I realized that my diagnosis was real.

Yes, this was all happening to me. But that didn't mean I didn't have faith, nor did it mean that I was unworthy or worthless because of a diagnosis. I had to remind myself that I was fearfully and wonderfully made[19] and that God had a

---

[19] Psalm 139:14.

purpose for the monkey wrench that was thrown in my life. To heal, I realized I would have to complete the cycles of grief.

Stage 2: Pain & Guilt

This hurts, God. I can't bear this alone. I can't bear to see another friend of mine pregnant and feel as though You don't hear me. It is my fault that I was diagnosed with infertility? If I'd never lost my virginity, I would be married by now and able to have kids. If I'd never been molested, my body would not have been thrown into perimenopause. If I'd never dated that guy, you told me not to date, maybe I wouldn't be here.

Pain and guilt had me thinking all sorts of crazy narratives about my fertility journey that weren't true. Above, I've written a few of the thoughts I had when going through this stage of grief. Can you relate to any of the statements listed? There were also the pity parties I had for myself, which led me into deep depression. I thought, *why should I even try to live? No one will marry me because I am broken. No man wants to marry a woman who can't bear him children.* False. False. False. It took me a while to navigate through pain and guilt. I want to repeat that it took me a while to navigate through pain and guilt. There isn't a timeline for how long this stage (or any of the stages for that matter) will last.

For me, this stage was the hardest to get through. On some days, the pain of the realization of what was going on with my body was gut-wrenching. I was an accomplished woman of God, but I couldn't control what my body was doing, which was disappointing and devastating. I did not have control. I could not fix it. I could not do it on my own.

Once I realized that I truly needed Jesus to perform a miracle, I surrendered my pain to him. God has a funny way of reminding us of His power, love, faithfulness, and character. I remember literally screaming at the top of my lungs on many nights as a way of expressing all my feelings to God. Honestly, Abba wants to hear from us even if all we know to do is yell. He wants to know how we're feeling.

After one of my screaming episodes, I received an email from one of the ministers at my church with a prayer for my spouse and children. I began to weep uncontrollably because it was a reminder that God heard my cries, knew my heart, and loved me unconditionally. My journey may be different from yours, but I want to remind you that God is faithful. God loves you, and He will get you through this.

Stage 3: Anger & Bargaining

I felt a sense of entitlement. I was a pastor's kid. I was smart, beautiful, talented, strong, and independent. Why would God do this to me? I didn't deserve this. I deserved to have everything my heart desired, right? That's what He promised me, right?

I remember getting angry with God. Yes, that's right, I got angry with God. Why? Because I felt like my life should go the way *I'd* planned it. Being thirty-four and unmarried was not in the plan. Infertility was not on my radar, and I should not have to go through it. I felt like God forsook me.

All the prayers I'd prayed over the years had gone in one ear and out the other. I asked God how He could take my biological mother *and* prevent me from becoming a mother myself. It just wasn't fair. I saw many women around me become blessed with children. Some were married and others were unmarried.

While I was happy for their blessing, I was hurt that God allowed the unmarried ones to conceive. I mean, I was taught that being pregnant out of wedlock is against His will, isn't it? Although I knew I wasn't perfect, at least I was *trying* to live a holy life. I deserved to be a wife. I deserved to be a mother.

I was not being unreasonable. Why did I have to wait? Why did I have to be chosen to be an example? I didn't want to be an example. Not in this way. God knew these were the only two things I ever wanted in life. Why would He do this to me?

I remember being so mad at God that I didn't want to go to church. Why? Because God wasn't answering my prayers. Through my angry tears, I couldn't see Jesus. I started losing my way and spiraling tremendously.

I was completely out of order, but I was being honest with my Creator. I was being honest because I knew He was listening. Now, did I have a complete two-year-old temper tantrum? Absolutely. But like any good parent, He let me have my moment before He began to speak to me. God reminded me of His love and asked me whether that was enough.

Was His love not greater than that of having a husband or being a mother? This is when I realized that I'd idolized marriage and motherhood. My actions broke God's heart. My reaction to my problem during the anger and bargaining stage of grief didn't catch God off guard, but it did disappoint Him. To me, there is nothing worse than disappointing God.

I had a constant battle of wills. Even though I was mad at God, I still prayed. There was still a little glimmer of hope mixed with a lot of desperation. During this season of my life, I was dating a guy and believed he was going to be my husband. When the first of January arrived, he still didn't know whether he wanted to be more than just friends, so I let him go. In rebellion and with the yearning to fill a void, I started seeing a guy I knew I should not have dated.

We were both toxic to each other. I was unstable, and he was bipolar. Eventually, there was a total explosion. Although we both believed in God and prayed together, we were not compatible. I overlooked *a lot* of red flags to be with him. There were things I knew I desired in a mate that he did not possess. For the sake of having a companion and trying to create a baby the right way since, in my mind, God wasn't going to do it for me, I stayed with him.

I call this the "Rebekah syndrome." Rebekah was told that Jacob would rule over his twin brother, Esau, even though Esau was the oldest. Instead of allowing God to work that thang right on out, she decided to take matters into her own hands, which ultimately made things worse.[20] In my anger and frustration, I made things way worse. I knew the guy I was dating wasn't the mate for me the day he told me that he didn't like the idea of being around family.

Although he had a son, he didn't like family because there were many issues in his family. He also didn't like holidays. Anyone who knows me knows that I love family, especially during the holidays. But because I wanted to start a family so badly, I stayed in the relationship and tried to make it work. I endured emotional and verbal abuse for about six months and tried to make it work even after he broke up with me.

Then one day, while scrolling on Facebook, I noticed that he posted something to the effect that he had a girlfriend even though we were still discussing reconciling the night before. When I called him out on it, he stated that it was a joke. Well, I let him know that I didn't find it funny and began to cut him off at that point. I blocked him on social media and began to heal from his toxicity. About a week later, he called to apologize.

---

[20] Gen. 27.

During his apology, he began flipping the blame on me. Yep, this hot mess of a relationship was because he was a narcissist. At that point, I was over it. I got quiet on the phone and said goodbye. I still wished him well and prayed that his relationship worked out, but I was done.

We hung up, and I blocked his number. I haven't spoken to him since. At some point during the relationship, I prayed that God would remove him from my life if he wasn't the one. Although it hurt, God came through and rescued me. I am so glad I serve a good, good Father who didn't let me stay in an unhealthy relationship. *El Roi* (a Hebrew name for God) saw me and delivered me out of the darkness of the hole I had dug for myself.

He reminded me of His love through my family, friends, and my village. I am forever grateful to God that I didn't stay in that relationship or the anger and bargaining stage of grief. I still prayed and fought while in my anger because I knew that God was still God. He is sovereign even on my worst days.

Stage 4: "Depression," Reflection, Loneliness

To me, this stage of grief is the hardest one. Depression is something that I wouldn't wish on anyone. No one should have to feel it, ever. The sunken place for me was just like it was portrayed in Jordan Peele's *Get Out*. In this movie, the main character is hypnotized and appears to begin to sink within himself, then he falls into a deep black hole of subconsciousness. That's what depression was for me. It felt like a never-ending, slow-motion descent into the unknown.

I had no joy or peace. I wanted to be left alone because I had no hope. I felt defeated, deflated, and dejected. There was no life in my eyes. All the things that I loved to do, I no longer enjoyed doing. I didn't want to sing. I didn't want to go to Zumba. I didn't want to leave my house. I had to literally press my way through this stage. It felt like the worst period of my life. I wanted to die. I thought about killing myself.

I mean, I thought that I no longer had purpose. I thought that God had abandoned me, and there were even days when I thought He didn't love me. Even though I was surrounded by love, I didn't actually feel it. It was hard to be motivated to do anything, especially look for a job. I was at my lowest of lows—my darkest of dark days. I was ready to give up.

One Sunday in between services, I was going into the choir room, as most praise teams and musicians do, to hang out and prepare for service. The drummer looked at me and asked, "Are you OK?" I was honest this day and told him I wasn't, but I didn't go into details as to what was going on. I went on into service and mustered up what strength I could to sing as I had done many Sundays before. When I sang, there was no feeling. I couldn't feel God; the Holy Spirit wasn't ministering through me. I was going through the motions just to make it through the day.

Not only was I depressed because of what I was dealing with, but my hormones were all out of whack as I mentioned earlier. So, the emotional and chemical sides of depression were working in harmony to keep me down, but I didn't stay there: "If the Son therefore shall make you free, ye shall be free indeed."[21] I had a host of people praying for me. I began to pray for myself again, then I released it. I gave it up, and that's when God blessed me.

Depression is common worldwide, and it is estimated that nearly seven percent of American adults have depression yearly. More than sixteen percent of U.S. adults—

---

[21] John 8:36 (KJV).

around one in six—will experience depression in their lifetime.[22]

If you are experiencing any of the following, please reach out and get help.

- Feeling very sad, hopeless, or worried
- Not enjoying things that used to give you joy
- Being easily irritated or frustrated
- Eating too much or too little
- Experiencing changes in how much you sleep
- Having a difficult time concentrating or remembering things
- Experiencing physical problems like headaches, stomachaches, or sexual dysfunction
- Thinking about hurting or killing yourself [23]

---

[22] Cleveland Clinic. "Depression: Types, Symptoms, Causes & Treatment," n.d. https://my.clevelandclinic.org/health/diseases/9290-depression.

[23] Cleveland Clinic. "Depression: Types, Symptoms, Causes & Treatment," n.d. https://my.clevelandclinic.org/health/diseases/9290-depression.

You are not alone. There are people who will pray with and for you and walk with you through your journey. If you ever find yourself thinking about suicide, please call **988** for the Suicide and Crisis Lifeline.

Stage 5: The Upward Turn

There is light at the end of the tunnel, and for me, I found myself again. It was March of 2019 when I finally felt my first release from grief. The grief cycle contains several stages, so you may revisit all or some stages many times depending on your trigger(s). The trick is to not stay where you are. The first time I knew that there was hope was after the annual women's conference at my church.

There, I shared my story publicly for the first time. We were doing an inspirational fashion show and each model's testimony was being read as she walked the runway. We were instructed to write our testimonies on a 3x5 notecard, and I used every inch of mine. The ladies heard my story, most for the first time, as I modeled a navy blue floral high low satin gown. It was a big deal for me because, at that time, I had been going through a season of self-shaming because I was the heaviest, I'd ever weighed in my entire life.

I also felt heavy spiritually because of all the pain I carried. I was uncomfortable in my skin and my clothes. The dress I wore was a size twelve, so at five feet and one inch, I was 160 pounds and lacked confidence just about every day. This may not seem significant to most, but when you're accustomed to being between 120-130 pounds, an extra thirty pounds can feel very uncomfortable.

On this day, I shared my story and walked out the back with my head held high because I was determined to be free. As I walked into the sanctuary from the choir room, I felt a sense of empowerment. Cheers and shouts of encouragement filled the room as I strutted my way to the pulpit. My friends, family, and other ladies in my church began to gas me up. As my story was being read out loud among strangers and loved ones for the first time, I couldn't hold my peace. I began to sob.

With my makeup done, hair looking cute, head held high, and confidence on deck, I broke down. Something about my story being read out loud made me feel naked and completely vulnerable. There was nothing I could do about it. There was nowhere to run or hide. The cat was out of the bag, and it was the most liberating thing ever.

My story of pain slowly became a journey of triumph. I believe it was at that moment that I decided I wasn't going to stay in my hole. I wanted out. I'm not sure if it was the fact that what I was going through was no longer a secret to the world or if it was the embrace my mother gave me after my fierce walk down the catwalk, but I knew I had a story to tell. I couldn't stay where I was.

I can't remember if it was that night or the next evening, but I recall going into my prayer/makeup room, turning off the lights, and lighting a candle. I began to pray. This time, it wasn't a cry to God asking why He allowed me to be fertility challenged. Rather, I thanked Him for trusting me with a calling. I repented for being disrespectful and angry with Him.

I repented for not trusting Him. I repented for doubting and disappointing Him. I began to ask Him to deliver me from depression and the victim syndrome I had been reveling in because I enjoyed the attention, I got from it. I asked God to restore my joy and show me the purpose in my season. I needed Him to help me get back on track so that I could fulfill His will for my life. I was coming out alive physically, spiritually, emotionally, and mentally.

Stage 6: Reconstruction and Working Through

The road to healing has not been an easy one. I received a breakthrough, but my healing process was just beginning. I still had days when I felt hopeless and down, but they began to be few and far in between. I was gifted a couple of therapy sessions. It felt great to be able to talk to someone about all I was going through.

Why didn't I go to my parents? You see, being a pastor's kid can be tricky at times. There are things that PKs see in the background that most church members don't. I didn't want to burden my parents with all that I was going through. I wasn't alone, but I also didn't want to overwhelm my parents either.

There was so much going on, but God. After going to therapy, having my mother take care of me (she insisted, of course), and experiencing my breakthrough at the conference, I began to take care of myself again. I started on a weight loss journey and moved out of my apartment. I created boundaries and safe spaces for myself, left my toxic ex in the past, and reignited my fire and passion for Christ. I got better day by day.

Were there setbacks? Of course! But the comebacks far outweighed the setbacks, so my hopelessness turned into hope. My faithlessness became faithfulness, and my heart that had been hardened began to soften again. I found myself reading my Word daily and making it a routine to pray at least once a day.

I began to change my priorities. I fasted from social media because sometimes scrolling was a trigger, and I made an effort to get out more. This by no means happened overnight. The process took time. Everyone's process is different, but this stage took me years to get through. Sometimes, I still revisit this stage depending on the trigger, but it has become much easier to get through. I truly began to embrace Philippians 4: 6-13. I learned how to be content when I had a lot and a little. I also realized that I could do all things through Christ who gives me strength.[24] I finally surrendered to the fact that God is in control and holds my future.

Stage 7: Acceptance & Hope

There's hope, and I am a living witness. One of the songs that got me through this season was "God's Gonna Do

---

[24] Phil. 4:13 (NLT).

It" by Ricky Dillard. On the way to church one Sunday, I was listening to the song and the Holy Spirit caught me. I was like, "Yes, Jesus! You're going to do it! Yes, God!"

When I reached the church parking lot, I immediately began shouting. This was during the pandemic. I was in the middle of purchasing a house and trying to get back in the dating game. I was enduring some challenges in both areas, but God. I began to declare that God was going to fulfill His promises to me.

God is not a man that He should lie, and I had to believe that. Why would He bring me this far just to leave me? So, I got a divorce. You read that right. I got a divorce. "Divorce" simply means to separate or dissociate from something. I came out of covenant with my idea of what my family would look like and began accepting what God had called me to be. What I was holding on to no longer served me any purpose. I was holding on to a fantasy, but not accepting my purpose, and this was holding me back from God's will for my life.

Divorcing my idea of what marriage and family should look like has been an entire roller coaster ride. I almost settled for being with a man who was not the right one for me to rush God's process. But like we see in the Bible with Sarah and Hagar or Rebekah with Jacob and Esau, we make more messes when we try to do things our way. If we just trust God, things will manifest according to His will and in His timing.

Why are we like this? Why do we make ourselves suffer unnecessarily? I didn't understand when my elders used to say to "just keep a living," but I understand it now. When God wants you to be somewhere or do something, you will be there and do that thing. God knows the plans He has for us. He orders our steps. He anoints and appoints us to be in places and carry burdens so that we can minister to others. Remember Paul and the thorn in his flesh?[25]

I have learned that this walk with God will not be the easiest, but it is made possible with Christ. I felt peace overtake me on the day that I finally settled in my spirit that this was my life. I was confident in knowing that the God of the universe always has my best interest in mind. Not only that, but I began to take the time to accept the season I was in and my calling to preach. I also accepted my calling to be a homeowner and an entrepreneur.

I began to heal internally and externally mend broken relationships. I apologized to others for bleeding on them because I was hurt and broken. I began to forgive others

---

[25] II Cor. 12: 6 - 10 (NLT).

because forgiveness is a huge part of healing. I started to become whole again. I felt renewed, free, and refreshed all because I let go and let God.

Remember that grief and healing are processes. You may repeat stages. You will have low days, but you will have high days as well. When you have a low day, you don't have to stay where you are. Do whatever it takes to not stay where you are. Phone a friend. Cry out to Jesus. Go to your favorite place. Go to therapy. See a professional. Do something that brings you happiness. Be determined to get out of that low place.

You must properly grieve because, if you don't, you will likely experience bitterness or hurt. You may also overcompensate, which might look like success, but it will catch up to you later and be more difficult to deal with. Trust me, I know. I've experienced this stage and have seen it happen with my own eyes. Please, if you have not grieved, take the time to do so properly.

Make it your mission to have the victory in this season of your life. Don't do it alone. Call upon your village to help you. God created them so that they could help you through your trying season. Doing so will help catapult you into your next season and give you room to live in your purpose.

My prayer for you:

Abba, please heal my dear sister's broken heart from any grief she may feel as she mourns the death of the way she thought things should be during her life's journey (Ps. 34:18).

Please give her the strength she needs today and every day to continue to pray and wait for the promise You made to her and her family (Phil. 4:13).

As she navigates throughout this process may she be reminded that she shouldn't be afraid because You are with her every step of the way (Ps. 23:4).

May you give her peace that surpasses all understanding in the moments where she is sobbing (Phil. 4:6 - 7), and may she feel your unspeakable joy in the moments where she feels her lowest (Ps. 28:7).

I ask that You remain her strength and that she will pull on You and rely on her family and friends to help her come out of this season victorious and filled with gratitude (Ps. 73:26). In Jesus' name I pray this prayer. Amen.

Chapter 6
Purpose in My Pain

And we know that all things work together for good to them that love God, to them who are the called according to his purpose.

–Romans 8:28 (KJV)

When I was diagnosed with perimenopause and pre-ovarian failure, I was unaware and uninformed, so I became scared, disappointed, and confused. I wondered, *How could this happen to me, God? Why me?* Then, the Lord said to me, "Why not you?" April 29, 2021, was day 277 since my last cycle. To be in full-fledged menopause, I had to go 365 days without having a cycle.

I was on day 277. I am not sure what prompted me to look at the app that tracked my cycle. For some odd reason, I decided to check it that day. As I opened the app, the number 277 glared at me as if it was saying, "HEEEEEEEEEYYYY, GIRL!!!" At that moment, I completely lost it. In my mind, menopause was about to become a reality, and I couldn't handle it. I began to ugly cry almost to the point of hyperventilating. I was a mess. I thought, *What are we doing, God? Am I about to go through this for real?*

I remember posting this message in the Womb Prep Facebook support group about the emotions I was having that day.

> **Ladies, today was rough for me. Today, I cried UGLY tears. Today, I realized it's been 277 days since my last period. That means that, according to science, menopause will be official in 88 days at the ripe age of 37. I cried . . . I'm still crying . . . I am not ok . . . I do not feel encouraged . . . I am still unmarried . . . I am still not pregnant . . . I need prayers . . . Today was not a good day.**

In the previous chapter, I mentioned that grief was cyclical and a process. There are days when you may return to one of the stages of grief that you thought you had overcome. One of those days for me was April 29, 2021. I cried and cried and cried. If it wasn't for the outpouring of love that I felt that day—the prayers, comments, texts, and calls—that were made by strangers and those I loved and knew, I know I would have completely given up on life. It was simply amazing.

Through my tears, hurt, disappointment, anguish, and fear, God sent a village to encourage me. I woke up on April 30th feeling better and more encouraged than the day before. I also made a conscious decision not to wallow in my sadness. I had to get up. I had work to do for God, and I had work to do as an employee and a business owner. May 1st was a working Saturday for me. I woke up before the sun.

If you know me, you know I am not a morning person. But regardless of how I felt, I made my way to Newnan, Georgia. A tornado had ravaged the town, so the local high school students weren't able to have their senior prom like usual. On top of the COVID-19 pandemic still going strong, the tornado further wrecked the plans for the prom. About eleven makeup artists (including myself) and roughly fifteen hairstylists from around Newnan and the metro Atlanta area volunteered our services for the young ladies who could not have the full prom experience. As I made my way to Newnan,

I thought about my body's changes and began to accept my menopausal fate.

I decided, again, that I would accept whatever God had in store for me. I wasn't going to be fearful. I would have complete faith that God would keep His promises to me. When I arrived at Newnan, I had to use the restroom after the two-hour drive. As I pulled up to the boarded up storefront church, I was greeted by some amazing souls who directed me to the restroom. (Disclaimer: I am about to be really transparent.) As I went to flush the toilet, I saw that the water was a little pink tinted. God started my cycle! Every time you have a cycle, you lose eggs, so I was conflicted in my emotions. I had a cycle, so I celebrated because I was no longer as close to menopause as I thought.

But having my cycle meant that I lost eggs. I cried all over again. This time, they were happy tears because I chose to praise God that I was no longer about to enter menopause. The whole ordeal was crazy because I'd put on a reusable pad because my vaginal area had been getting embarrassingly musty. I thought the pad would help to control the odor. By doing that, I was already prepared to handle what God had coming my way that day. I couldn't wait to tell the Womb Prep tribe and my bestie what God had done for me. That day, I started back at day one and posted this in the group:

> ***PRAISE REPORT!!! Ladies! Ladies! Ladies! I just want to tell y'all that the tears I'm crying today are tears of joy. I want to thank all of y'all from the bottom of my heart for all y'all prayers. Day 279 . . . My cycle came . . . Y'all, I want to cry ugly tears but can't right now because I'm in public. I love y'all!!!***

Again, there was an outpouring of praise and adoration to God for His goodness and blessing upon me. God used me in that moment to show His power, and He did so mightily. Through that act, God revealed even more that there was literally purpose in my pain. After my diagnosis, I was eager to begin advocating for women like myself, professional and unmarried without children, to take the time to learn about their bodies and their ability to have children before it is too late. To do this, I began the Motherhood Foundation, Inc.

I wanted to provide scholarships for women who wanted to have in vitro fertilization (IVF) or adopt. Also, I wanted to lead workshops, have a fashion show, and do so much more. I even started applying for grants, but I stopped because I discovered that the direction, I was going in was not the one

God had for me. Although I was getting the word out about the foundation, I had a lot of losses in 2019. In 2020, I began to make plans for the Motherhood Foundation to recoup what had been lost in 2019.

I recruited a few of my sister-friends to help me promote the Mind Your Own Uterus™ campaign. I shared the stories of women who were experiencing infertility and why it was so important to not ask a woman about her fertility status. I planned to educate people on good conversation starters that would exclude any topics surrounding fertility and even got T-shirts made. But, before any of my plans could get off the ground, COVID-19 hit and shut down production. Allowing myself to bounce back, I took to social media and pivoted.

I started (and continue) to promote my Mind Your Own Uterus™ campaign, and T-shirts are still available at *www.allthingsalishaj.com*. Instead of desiring to only grow myself, I decided that I would bring others with me. I continue to educate and raise awareness about infertility, knowing one's status, and minding one's own uterus. My journey has shown me that my purpose is multilayered. Back in September of 2020, I awoke in the middle of the night to a hot flash. Although this had become my norm, on this particular night, I decided to do something different. I began to pray.

I prayed for women who were going through infertility journeys and fertility challenges. I made this a habit moving forward and affectionately called them the "hot flash prayers." I took this even further by posting about my purpose on Facebook and praying for others whenever I had a hot flash. This was the original post:

> *I'm turning my PAIN into PRAYER. Most of you know my story concerning the diagnosis of infertility. I say "the diagnosis" because I am no longer claiming it as mine. I believe in God's miraculous healing power, and I know that God is allowing me to experience this for a reason. Although, it may be a hard pill to swallow at times (real talk), I know that God's Word is true and that all things work together for my good (Romans 8:28). With that said, I will rejoice in all things and use my story to minister to others. From now until my birthday, I am committing to pray for someone for every hot flash that wakes me up in the middle of the night. If you have any prayer*

requests, please DM (direct message) me, and I will commit to praying for you during at least one of those instances. Love you all. Remember that God is a MIRACLE WORKER!

Even now, I still whisper prayers for others when I have a hot flash from time to time. It may not be every time, but I remind myself to pray. This season of my life has had some amazing highs and some devastating lows, but God has been there through it all. I have been more purposeful in spending time with God, learning how to pray, praying more, and being more intentional about how I maximize my time with the people I love and things that I enjoy doing. I've been more about YOLO (you only live once) than being as overly cautious as I once was (I'm still living holy and fulfilling the purpose God has for my life). I have to check my feelings every day.

With every baby or proposal announcement, I've had to learn how to properly address my feelings of sadness by focusing on the happiness of the moment and counting the blessings I have as opposed to comparing my lack of being pregnant to someone else's abundance thereof. I've also changed the way I look at proposals and baby announcements. I began affirming myself. For every announcement, I declare "I'm next" and keep scrolling.

I began turning my pain into victory by focusing on what God promised me. The song by Ricky Dillard that I referenced in the previous chapter has been helping me get through this season. I suggest that you find yourself a good song to minister to your soul and get you through. It helps so much. In this particular song, the lead ad libs "God made me a promise. I still believe in God." The Bible declares that God is not a man that He should lie.[26]

He made me a promise, and I believe His promises. That is the hope that I hold onto. This may not be the case for you, but He sent three different prophets who had no idea about my situation to assure me that I would give birth. Even in the midst of me writing this book, I've been blessed and will continue to give God glory because I know that I will be a mother in His time. The next book I will write will chronicle God's fulfillment of His promises to me.[27]

---

[26] Num. 23:19.

[27] Isa. 60:22.

My prayer for you:

Abba, I pray that as my dear sister is going through her life's journey that she will find the purpose in all the pain she has experienced. Whether it be from the loss of a relationship that she thought was going to end in marriage or a diagnosis of infertility (Prov. 16:9).

I pray that she will find peace in You and that she will fully depend on You to get her through the tough seasons of her life (Ps. 23:1).

I pray that she will not feel alone, but know that You are with her, guiding her every step of the way, renewing her strength along the way (Ps. 23:3).

May she fear no evil because You, Abba, are with her, even in the darkest valley (Ps. 23:4).

Please grant her wisdom (James 1:5) and may she dream dreams and have visions concerning the purpose in her pain (Acts 2:17) so that what she is going through may be a blessing to others and a testament of your faithfulness (Lam. 3:22 – 23). In Jesus' name I pray this prayer. Amen.

Chapter 7

The Village

Greater love has no one than this: to lay down one's life for one's friends.

–John 15:13 (NIV)

This book would be incomplete without mentioning that God has blessed me with an amazing village of people who prayed and helped me navigate this journey. My path has been more bearable because of God and all the people I surrounded myself with. There is no way I would have made it this far without them. Every woman or couple should have a solid village to help them through their season of infertility because it makes a world of difference. Whether they are people to rally around you in prayer, raise funds for you, be a listening ear when you're having a low moment, or take you out of the house, a village is an essential resource to aid you throughout your journey to motherhood.

My parents have been my rocks. Amid all the things going on in their personal lives, they were there for me. Their love and care supported me through all my pain and disappointment. Even when I was a brat, my parents still helped me. When going through this journey, make sure you have people who will be your rock. My parents prayed with me, encouraged me, and physically took care of me during my battle with depression. They welcomed me back home when I had to move out of my apartment and let me stay long enough to get back on my feet. I know without a shadow of a doubt that I would not be where I am now without my amazing parents.

My village also includes a terrific team of doctors who encouraged and prayed for me. As a black Christian woman, it is so important to me to have a team of doctors who look like me and believe the same things I do. The way that my doctors have cared for me has been unorthodox but such a blessing. My doctors prayed for and with me, felt my disappointments, and encouraged me along the way. They look out for me still today because of the relationship that I have with them. When you are on this journey, having the right medical care team makes a world of difference. You need professionals that will treat you more like family than like a patient. It not only helps you go through your process, but it helps strengthen your faith.

Medical professionals who believe like you believe are important, but it is a bonus to have a Christian therapist to help you navigate the stages of grief mentioned before. There is nothing wrong with having Jesus and therapy. I would also like to thank my therapist for being a listening ear and providing practical, spiritual guidance while I navigate this season.

Additionally, I would like to call out my aunt, Nancy Blanding, for accompanying my mother to one of my many doctor visits. When I told my aunt about my fibroid issue, she paid special attention and made it her mission to research fibroids. She and my Uncle Vincent were integral parts of my prayer warrior team, along with my godmother, Auntie Myra Jones, countless other family members, my bestie, Nicole Carter, and many close friends. All of those who have been on this roller coaster ride with me know me intimately, know my temperament, and know how to minister to me and love on me when I need it the most. I didn't let a lot of people know about my situation until that day at the fashion show. I knew that I could trust my village with my journey, and I knew they would be there support me no matter what.

During this season, I was introduced to Geri Alicea, who has an infertility journey of her own. Our mutual friend, Brandi, interviewed Geri during National Infertility Week, which is the third week of April.

After watching the Facebook Live, I was drawn to Geri, so I went on Facebook and stalked her a little. While doing my research, I discovered her book, *The Journey to Motherhood*, and her Facebook support group, Womb Prep, which I later joined. I couldn't believe how many other women were like me. I had no idea that there were even support groups for us. Geri's book not only helped me to heal, but the online community she founded encourages me even to this day. It's a true sisterhood.

Soon after finishing her book, I invited Geri to be a guest on my radio show, *Church Girl Reality*. Shortly after, we bonded and now co-host the *Journey to Motherhood* podcast (available wherever podcasts are heard). One of our podcast episodes speaks to the importance of having a support system. It truly is a blessing when you don't have to go through a trial or tribulation alone. So, I encourage you to surround yourself with people who will pray for you and uplift you on your journey. Know that you are not alone. There are millions of women who are in your shoes and more than willing to lend a listening ear and a compassionate heart.

My prayer for you today:

Abba, I pray that my sister has a strong village like I do, who loves her, who is rooting for her, and who wants her to live out her wildest dreams (John 15: 12 – 13).

May they pray for her more than she prays for herself and may she feel the prayers of those who love her (Job 16: 20 – 21).

If she doesn't have a support system, I pray that she knows that I am here for her and that there is a tribe of ladies who will pray and believe for and with her for her future husband and children, for the prayers of the righteous avails much (James 5:16).

Please surround her with love today and all the days of her life so that she can remain motivated and peaceful while on her journey to marriage and motherhood (I Cor. 13). In Jesus' name I pray this prayer. Amen.

Chapter 8
Don't Put Your Eggs in One Basket

The steps of a good man are ordered by the Lord: and he delighteth in his way.

–Psalm 37:23 (KJV)

    The journey to motherhood is different for everyone, especially if you have challenges along the way. I wrote this book in hopes of encouraging women of color, who are spending most of their twenties and thirties establishing their careers or building their businesses, to slow down for a moment to consider their options for motherhood before they are presented with challenges. First and foremost, please ask your OB-GYN to have the proper hormone tests done outside of your routine physical. Request that they test to see your levels and determine if you are close to menopause based on your current egg count. Second, while you are planning your future, make sure to plan for your family as well.

On average, black women are waiting until age thirty-two to marry.[28] At thirty-four, I thought I still had time to have children. Know your body more intimately and make sure you have the right OB-GYN who will listen to you when you say that you want to make sure your body is ready to carry and give birth to a child when the time is right. If you are where I am, still unmarried without children and facing fertility challenges or are currently married but facing infertility, please consider the following options with much prayer.

Adoption can be expensive and an emotional roller coaster from what I have been told. Outside of being able to adopt a child from within your own family, adoption can be expensive, starting at $15,000 if you are adopting from a private agency. The process itself can be very long based on whether you want to adopt as a married or single woman, and the availability of the child you want to adopt based on age,

---

[28] "Current Population Reports - Census.gov," accessed December 16, 2022, https://www.census.gov/content/dam/Census/library/publications/2021/demo/p70-167.pdf.

gender, ethnicity, etc. Additionally, most agencies do thorough background checks to ensure that you are a worthy candidate. So, your home must always be kept a certain way while you wait to be matched with your child. I have been told that depending on which state you reside in, the process for adoption differs, so I suggest doing research to assess your options.

Foster care is an option to care for a child temporarily while their main caregivers prepare to obtain full custody of the child again. In some cases, you may have the option to adopt the child. One of my guests on *Church Girl Reality* stated that being a foster parent is like miscarrying a child repeatedly. You are constantly having to detach yourself from a child that you've fallen in love with. I am telling you this not to discourage you from the foster care system but to prepare you emotionally for what may be in your future. Additionally, if you can adopt a child that you have fostered, the process may be less expensive. But again, I suggest that you consult your local laws to confirm your options.

Embryo adoption is the option to adopt an embryo, or a fertilized egg, from a family that has embryos from IVF that they don't plan on having implanted. Embryo adoption allows the genetic parents to give their embryos a chance for life.[29] Be mindful of having conversations to address your child's medical history and other genetic family matters. Prepare yourself if you go down this route. Although costly, this option may be less expensive than that of a normal adoption, starting at $10,000.

Egg freezing aka oocyte cryopreservation, consists of a woman's eggs being extracted, frozen, and stored for future use. The success rates are estimated between 4–12 percent, and the process costs around the same as embryo adoption.[30] From personal experience, this can be an emotional roller coaster because of all the hormone therapy that is involved, on top of the raw emotions that you will experience just going through the process. I suggest making sure you secure a village of people that will support you throughout this process, as it can be daunting to experience alone.

IVF is the joining of a woman's egg and a man's sperm in a laboratory dish. "In vitro" means outside the body.

---

[29] National Embryo Donation Center. "Adoption," n.d. https://embryodonation.org/adoption.

[30] UCLA Health. "Fertility and Reproductive Health - Egg Freezing," n.d. https://www.uclahealth.org/medical-services/obgyn/fertility/egg-freezing.

"Fertilization" means the sperm has attached to and entered the egg.[31] According to the *New York Times*, IVF is on average around $15,000-$17,000, not including the medication. With medication, the cost can rise to closer to $25,000. An IVF cycle is defined as one egg retrieval and all the embryo transfers that result from that retrieval.

Intrauterine insemination (IUI) is a type of artificial insemination where sperm are placed directly in your uterus around the time your ovary releases one or more eggs to be fertilized.[32] IUI, if not covered by insurance, can cost around $1,000. If you are unmarried, this does not include the cost of acquiring donor sperm. As with any procedure dealing with infertility, there are risks and emotional connections that you may face, so I recommend that you have a therapist or counselor lined up while going through this process.

Donor eggs come from a woman who gives her eggs to another woman (recipient) to allow her to have a baby. The eggs are removed from the donor by placing a needle that is attached to an ultrasound probe through the vaginal tissues.

---

[31] Medline Plus. "In vitro fertilization (IVF)," n.d. https://medlineplus.gov/ency/article/007279.htm.

[32] Mayo Clinic. "Intrauterine insemination (IUI)," September 03, 2021. https://www.mayoclinic.org/tests-procedures/intrauterine-insemination/about/pac-20384722.

The eggs are then gently aspirated (suctioned) from the ovaries.[33] Egg donation can start at $20,000.[34]

Donor sperm can cost anywhere between $400 to $2,000 if purchased from a sperm bank. Donor sperm can also come from a close relative or friend (hopefully) at no cost to you.[35]

I have provided brief descriptions of the few options that I am aware of currently, but please consult a medical professional to discuss which option(s) make more sense for you in this season. Don't forget to consult the ultimate physician, Abba Father, as He knows what is best for you and your future family.

In 2019, I attempted to freeze my eggs because I thought it was a good idea. Based on the circumstances, it was a good idea, but it wasn't a God idea. I realized I hadn't consulted God on how He wanted this story to unfold. I

---

[33] American Society for Reproductive Medicine. "Egg Donation," March 9, 2017. https://www.reproductivefacts.org/utility-container/search-results/?q=donor+eggs.

[34] Egg Bank America/Egg Donor America. "Egg Donor Fees and Costs," https://www.eggdonoramerica.com/parents/egg-donor-fees-costs.

[35] Forbes Health. "Sperm Donor Cost: What You Need to Know," November 2, 2022. https://www.forbes.com/health/family/sperm-donor-cost/.

honestly thought I was working my faith because faith without works is dead[36]. But we also know that some things only come by fasting and prayer[37]. For now, I will wait on God to perform this miracle His way. Adoption has always been something that I wanted to do, even before the diagnosis, so I am seeking God concerning this as well because I have heard that it can be simultaneously rewarding yet challenging.

However, God chooses for this journey to reveal His miracle, I am down for it, but I am prayerful concerning what direction as I wait for motherhood and the man, He set aside for me to marry. I believe the Word He has spoken over my life, and I receive it as well. In the meantime, I have recommitted to eating better, being more aware of the foods I ingest, exercising more, and taking care of myself spiritually, emotionally, mentally, and physically to prepare for the family that is coming.

I pray that you, too, will ask God for the direction you should go. This will not only save you from potential heartache, but it may also save you money. Also, make sure

---

[36] James 2:26 (NLT).

[37] Mark 9:29 (KJV).

your village is on board with you as you make your decisions concerning motherhood. Their support will be an integral part of your journey depending on your choice.

Whatever you do, don't give up on the promise God has for you, for at the right time, God will make it happen[38]. I also encourage you to research each of the options I mentioned earlier to see which one is best for you or consult your OB-GYN to refer you to a reproductive specialist. You can visit themotherhoodfoundation.com for more information about your options and possible scholarships available to you.

My pain has produced a purpose that I could have never imagined. Out of this, I have started a ministry, formed a business, and written a book. I am living my best life. My "rich aunty" phase has been activated. I am traveling more than I have ever done, enjoying the freedom to come and go as I please. I'm cooking for a party of one or not cooking at all if I don't feel like. I am also embracing that the only person I need to consult with at this point is God.

I am taking the time to take care of me, loving on myself and dating myself. I am also making sure that I am healed and whole before I completely open myself up to a

---

[38] Isaiah 60:22 (NLT).

man. This step is so important. My main focus is on myself and God, and I am truly content with being single. I know that God made me a promise, and He will come through for me. The same God that will do it for me will do it for you, too. No matter how long you have been single, God will come through for you. I encourage you to take up a hobby, travel the world, make new friends, invest in yourself, and learn who you are in God so that, when the time is right and the Lord makes it happen, you will be ready.

After reading this, I am praying that you will experience the freedom of your unmarried season and take God at His Word. Focus on yourself, preparing for marriage and learning how to navigate your fertility challenges or determine what fertility options the Holy Spirit is leading you to pursue in your season of waiting.

If you've never been to Aruba, I suggest you go. It is not in the hurricane belt, the water is crystal clear, and the people are kind. You never know who you will meet along the way!

If you're reading this book and need support, please reach out to me at *www.allthingsalishaj.com*. I'd love to connect with other women who are navigating their own journeys to marriage and motherhood. I am here for you—to pray for and agree with you that God will do it. You don't have to walk alone. Promise me that you won't let this season of your life be a period. Rather, make it a comma that is preparing you for what is to come.

Married With Children, loading...

My prayer for you:

Abba, as we bring this book to a close, I want to thank You for my sister and her journey to marriage and motherhood.

I pray that she enjoys her rich aunty life and that you will give her wisdom as she dates and explores her options to motherhood (Prov. 4:7).

May You work supernaturally in her life and give her a hope and a future (Jer. 29:11).

I ask that You bless her exceedingly and abundantly above all she could ask or think over her life, her future marriage, and her future children (Eph. 3:20).

Please keep her in perfect peace as she keeps her mind stayed on You (Isaiah 26:3) and may she walk by faith and not by sight (2 Cor. 5:7).

Last, but certainly not least, I pray that she doesn't become weary in well doing because in due season she

will reap what you promised her, if she does not lose heart (Gal. 6:9). In Jesus' name I pray this prayer. Amen.

Bibliography

"7 Stages of Grief - Going Through the Process and Back to Life." Recover from Grief. Last modified March 30, 2020. www.recover-from-grief.com/7-stages-of-grief.html.

"Anti-Müllerian Hormone Test." Medline Plus. Last modified December 15, 2020. https://medlineplus.gov/lab-tests/anti-mullerian-hormone-test/.

Editorial Committee IVI Blog. "What is a follicle and how many follicles do you need?" IVI. Last modified April 1, 2020.

https://ivi-fertility.com/blog/follicle-how-many-follicles-do-you-need/.

"Follicle-Stimulating Hormone (FSH) Levels Test." Medline Plus. Last modified December 17, 2020.

https://medlineplus.gov/lab-tests/follicle-stimulating-hormone-fsh-level s-test/.

Goldberg, Joanna. "Follicle-Stimulating Hormone (FSH) Test." Healthline. Last modified September 17, 2018.

https://www.healthline.com/health/fsh#purpose.

"Infertility FAQs." Centers for Disease Control and Prevention (CDC). Last modified March 1, 2020. https://www.cdc.gov/reproductivehealth/infertility/index.htm.

Mayol-Garcia, Yeris, Benjamin Gurrentz, and Rose M. Kreider. "Number, Timing, and Duration of Marriages and Divorces: 2016." *U.S. Department of Commerce* (April 2021): 70-167.

"Ovarian cysts - Symptoms and Causes." Mayo Clinic. Last modified 2022. https://www.mayoclinic.org/diseases-conditions/ovarian-cysts/sympto ms-causes/syc-20353405.

"Sharing Our Story – A Conversation About Infertility in the Black Community." Resolve. Last modified March 5, 2021. https://resolve.org/sharing-our-story-a-conversation-about-infertility-in- the-black-community/.

"Uterine fibroids - Symptoms and Causes." Mayo Clinic. Last modified 2022. https://www.mayoclinic.org/diseases-conditions/uterine-fibroids/sympt oms-causes/syc-20354288.

www.ingramcontent.com/pod-product-compliance
Lightning Source LLC
Chambersburg PA
CBHW022014160426
43197CB00007B/427